GROW THE HEALTH UP

Lauren

Thank you!
for your support and
you health

Wishing
and Wellness

GROW THE HEALTH UP

Healthy Living Creates Healthy Lives

Debra McLemore Duffy

GROW THE HEALTH UP
Copyright 2020 Debra McDuffy

Some names of persons mentioned in this book have been changed to protect privacy. Any similarities between individuals described in this book to individuals known to readers are purely coincidental.

Printed in the United States of America

Hardback ISBN 978-1-7356773-0-1
Paperback ISBN 978-1-7356733-1-8
eBook ISBN 978-1-17356733-2-5

Scripture marked KJV are ataken from the KING JAMES VERSION (KJV); KING JAMES VERSION, public domain.

Scripture marked NIV and NIV 85 taken from New International Version (NIV): Scripture taken from Thee HOLY BIBLE,

NEW INTERNATIONAL VERSION, Copyright 1973, 1978, 1989, 2011 by Biblica, Inc; Used by permission of Zondervan

Contents

DEDICATION

I was born for the purpose of spreading the word about God, faith, fitness and health. Thank you, God, for trusting me to spread your word about the stewardship of our temples. When I look back over my life, I clearly see your hands, God.

My parents, being my first teachers of how to walk this earth with grace and purpose, are a priceless example of what to do and how to do it. They understand the foundation of *legacy*. From them I learned to *lead by example*. I learned *do not talk about it, do not give illustrations; just do it.*

My earliest memory of having an "aha" moment about life's obstacles was when I was eight years old living in Germany with my family. I enjoyed running, jumping, sports, and dancing. I remember having a rough time getting over a branch that was on the ground in our back yard. I told my parents how hard it was to jump over the branch and that it was hard to stop thinking about it. My mother said, "Hard is hard." It took me until I was in my twenties to understand that statement. What I have come to understand is if I desire to do something, like writing this book, it is going to be hard because I am not the best scholar. It has been hard sitting back the past two years thinking about it every day.

When faced with hard decisions, leap anyway. Hard is not the objective. The real objective is to leave a legacy of jumpers who will not consent to obstacles stopping them. They recognize the branches they will face may slow their pace, but will not keep them from their destiny. The branches that get in your way will not be the hardest thing you will ever get over.

Thank you, Mom and Dad, for the "heart" lesson.

ACKNOWLEDGEMENTS

This book is one I believe God summoned me to write at this time. I thank Him for trusting me to use my voice to help others learn how to have a healthier life experience. I would be remiss if I did not acknowledge my ever patient husband and children. Our journey together has been filled with life's ups and downs, but through it all, we have never abandoned our idea of living life to the fullest.

Thank you to my husband, Retired LTC Jerome C. Duffy, Jr., for providing a lifestyle of safety to our family. As a military family, we have been called often to regulate our daily movement. We take pride in being ambassadors representing the best America has to offer, while having boots on the ground and living abroad. We realize better than most about not leaving a "wounded warrior behind." We are led by faith that our lives are bigger than our family and that we are to serve the least of them.

Thank you to my daughters, Brianna, Danielle, and Juanita, for being my reason to maintain a healthy lifestyle. Thank you for helping me during my many fitness sessions, health seminars, classes, and for your unwavering support. When God made girls, he gave me the best!

Thank you to Jordan and Arianna for coming into my life. You gave me the courage to accept my flaws and you pushed me to grow.

To my grandbabies, you may not realize this right now, but I am grateful for you because you represent forgiveness in my life.

Thank you, Abby. God illustrated His Grace for me through you!

Margo, thank you for being one of my biggest cheerleaders, May you R.I.H.

God, I give you thanks in everything. I give God the glory for His mercy even during the times of renewing my spirit.

FOREWORD

I grew up during the era that even when life got busy, fast food was *not* the go-to option. If we went to a restaurant it was because it was a special occasion. Although my siblings and I were given a menu, we knew hamburgers and fries were not an option for us. We understood our parents paid for the meals. Our parents recognized that a well-balanced meal meant we would not come back in a couple hours saying we were hungry or that we wanted a snack. To be honest, parents back then did not go for eating dinner and then eating more food later. Their economic status did not support such behavior.

Much has been written about weight loss, obesity, and exercise. I challenge you to take a step back and talk about a legacy of living well. You may have heard the saying, "Eat to live, not live to eat." That seems to be easier said than done. We are at the threshold of *replace* or *repair* rather than prevention. It is acceptable to announce that you are suffering from illnesses such as high blood pressure, diabetes, and dementia, yet your social circle or even family and friends will invite you over for a barbecue with all the trimmings. At work, there is always a reason to eat. The selection is usually unhealthy, and you can go back and get as much as you like. Here is where you will hear phrases like "You only live once," "I only eat this in moderation," or "I'm going to die from something." I guess your friends and family support your choices. I get it; good food is food worth tasting, but at what expense.

I task you to have the conversation with your children about how different foods can affect the body. Explain how food is necessary for building your body. This not only adds a richer, deeper, and more meaningful reason to be faithful to your physical body, but it opens your spiritual eyes as to why you should take care of your temple (body).

"I beseech you therefore, brethren, by the mercies of God, that ye present your bodies a living and holy sacrifice, acceptable to God, which is your reasonable service. And be not conformed to this world: but be ye transformed by the renewing of your mind, that ye may prove what is that good, and acceptable, and perfect, will of God" (Romans 12:1-2 KJV).

The Background

EVERYTHING IN LIFE HAS A PURPOSE

My earliest memory of health and wellness started when I was around eight years old and in the second grade. My father was in the military. We were living in Wurzburg, Germany at the time. Mrs. Schmitz, my teacher, had the class do an experiment using a jar with a lid, a piece of meat, and a can of soda pop. The instructions were for each student to 1) place the meat inside the jar, pour the soda pop into the jar, 3) place the lid on the jar, 4) place the jar on the classroom counter, and 5) do not open the jars for five days.

Each day, almost as soon as I walked into the classroom, I checked on my jar. The first twenty-four hours after putting the meat and pop into the jar, I noticed the color of the meat changed from a pretty pink to a dull maroon. By day three, the meat was dark brown. Most of the soda pop had absorbed into the meat and the meat was drying out. Mrs.

Schmitz told us to put a hole in the top of our jars. When we did this, the air in the classroom filled with a horrible smell. It was so bad we had to open the windows. On day five, the last day of the experiment, we removed our lids. The meat was completely black and the odor was indescribable. We took our piece of meat out of our jars. The meat was hard and had a rubbery feel to it. At the time, I remember thinking if drinking soda pop smelled like this, and could do something like this to the inside of my body, then I wanted no parts of it. Do not get me wrong; the experiment did not keep me from drinking pop. It did, however, set the tone for me to live as healthy as possible.

I am now aware that Mrs. Schmitz was teaching us that the liver is the conductor for removing harmful toxins out of the body. It is like having a filter that keeps debris out of your bloodstream. It is fascinating that the liver was made to produce hormones, blends to allow for proper digestion, and stores energy. Later, I will discuss how food is used for either energy or fat, but not both.

There has been an increasing concern among health professionals, and the like, about problems we face with the healthcare system. The state of our overall health in America, especially for young children, is concerning. Many families are finding themselves in a state of emergency as it relates to health. According to Centers for Disease Control (CDC) and Prevention, data from 2014 show nearly 1 in 5 school age children and young people (6 to 19 years) in the United States have obesity. Obesity is defined as having excess body fat. Body fat is measured using the Body Mass Index (BMI). The Health industry is a billion dollar business. Yet, we are still seeking solutions rather than using preventive methods to decrease expanded waistlines, diseases and illnesses.

Movement and nutrition are two of the most important things to human survival. Many people struggle with both. One would think this would not be a challenge to people in this *advanced* world. We are indeed embarking on a malnutrition era and muscle atrophy state. Most people already know what it will take to live a healthier lifestyle. One school of thought is to eat six small meals, cut out saturated fat, increase daily intake of fruits and vegetables, drink at least 64 ounces of water daily, and reduce meat and sweets. Couple this with 30-45 minutes of exercise 3-5 days a week.

11 *And the LORD shall guide thee continually, and satisfy thy soul in drought, and make fat thy bones: and thou shalt be like a watered garden, and like a spring of water, whose waters fail not. 12 And they that shall be of thee shall build the old waste places: thou shalt raise up the foundations of many generations; and thou shalt be called, The repairer of the breach, The restorer of paths to dwell in. Isaiah 58: 11-12KJV*

BMI = BODY MASS INDEX

Underweight ....Less than 19

Healthy weight 19-24.9

Overweight 25-29.9

Obese... ....Greater than 30

TARGET HEART RATE ZONE

Target heart rate measures the amount of effort used during any given exercise. Taking your pulse will help you to monitor or gauge if you need to decrease the intensity or increase the intensity of output/work that you are putting into your workout. Find your target zone for your age group. Example, for a 22 year-old the target zone is 138-168 bpm.

Target Heart Zone Formula	220-22 (age) = 198 bpm
Calculating Moderate Heart Rate of Maximal heart rate X 70% Equals threshold heart rate	198 bpm X.70 138 bpm (135.6)
Calculating High-Max Heart Rate of Maximal heart rate x 85% Equals threshold heart rate	198 bpm x.85 168 bpm (168.3)

The question is how we can achieve this with our busy lifestyles. By writing down what you're doing. Diagrams A and B will give you a how-to guide to start a physical weight training program.

UPPER BODY EXERCISES DATE:

Chest: *Exercise/choose one from each group*	Reps	Weight Lifted	Notes
SM Incline Press DB Bench Press Military Press Pushups	X X X X		
Back: *Exercise/choose one from each group*	Reps	Weight Lifted	Notes
Low Row Mid Row Lat Pull (towards the back) Pullover One Arm DB	X X X X X		
Shoulders: *Exercise/choose one from each group*	Reps	Weight Lifted	Notes
DB Shoulder Press Front Raises Lateral Raises	X X X		
Biceps: *Exercise/choose one from each group*	Reps	Weight Lifted	Notes
Alternative DB Curls Preacher Curls Bicep Curls Cable Curls	X X X X		
Triceps: *Exercise/choose one from each group*	Reps	Weight Lifted	Notes
SM Triceps Ext Triceps Ext (DB) Triceps Cable Ext	X X X		

Try increasing your weight on each set, but never sacrifice your body position.

5

Diagram B: One way to journal what you are doing is to log each time you perform any of the Lower Body Exercises.

LOWER BODY EXERCISES DATE:

Quadriceps: Exercise/ choose one from each group	Reps	Weight Lifted	Notes
Leg Press	X		
Quad Extension	X		
Squats	X		
Multi-Hip	X		
Hamstrings: Exercise/ choose one from each group	Reps	Weight Lifted	Notes
Leg Press	X		
Quad Extension	X		
Squats	X		
Prone Curls	X		
Lunges	X		
Gluteus: Exercise/choose one from each group	Reps	Weight Lifted	Notes
Gluteus	X		
Buster	X		
Inner/Outer	X		
Thigh/Multi-Hip	X		
Abs: Exercise/choose one from each group	Reps	Weight Lifted	Notes
Floor Crunches	X		
Oblique's Crunches	X		
Reverse Crunches	X		
Hanging Knee Raises	X		

Try increasing your weight on each set, but never sacrifice your body position.

What if I told you that you can change the course of the health of your children and their children with one decision? Would you be interested?

Ask yourself, how do I measure up in this era of mental health? When negative thoughts come to your mind; how do you work through them?

_____

_____

_____

_____

_____

_____

_____

_____

_____

_____

_____

_____

Our first architect to building a body and mind of optimal health is God. Through His word we have been given a template to how we are to treat our temple, also known as the *body*. Mothers, fathers, and guardians can be instruments used to teach children how to achieve a healthy lifestyle over their lifespan. The role they play in wellness and prevention is reliant on a planned strategy to maintain a good quality of life. Mothers tend to set schedules for their children and even their spouses to follow. They have set times they want their kids to get up, to eat, time to do academic learning, and time to sleep. The phrase *"shake what your momma gave you"* is true during the infant to adolescent stages. During these stages, children rely on a parent/guardian to provide their needs and wants. Most of the time if a child is obese, and it is not due to medical reasons, it is due to the guidance of the parent(s), guardian, or caregiver.

When you are obese as an adult, it is usually based on the choices you have made, coupled perhaps with influence from early childhood decisions. If a mother (parent/caregiver) would look at health in the way that it is everlasting, and if they thought bad health is preventive, in most cases, why are they not being as proactive about prevention as they are about manicures, hair appointments, sports, buying clothes and shoes, arranging play dates, and scrapbooking, to name a few? The outer appearance has not been proven to be lasting. Those organs that could be used to save others' lives well after the spirit has passed should be healthy as possible.

Good parenting is often measured by how happy children appear to be at any given moment. There is a measuring stick for how *healthy* children appear to be at any given time. When leaning towards optimal health, it can be a challenge to get your child to eat nutritional foods rather than foods less favorable. As an option, one decision could be to become the creator of possibilities for your legacies (children).

If you are a parent or guardian of a child today, list six (6) healthiest behaviors you would pass on.

1. _____

2. _____

3. _____

4. _____

5. _____

6. _____

If you are a parent or guardian of a child today, list six (6) least healthiest behaviors you would pass on.

1. _____

2. _____

3. _____

4. _____

5. _____

6. _____

If you are a parent or guardian of a child today, list six (6) hereditary behaviors you would pass on from your maternal and paternal families.

1. _____

2. _____

3. _____

4. _____

5. _____

6. _____

This Relationship Is Fatigued!

Over your lifetime, you probably have experienced the need to end a relationship or you know of someone who has. At times, it may be easy to end a relationship. Other times, it can be one of the most difficult decisions to make and be present during the process. There are many ways to end a relationship. Some people may choose to write a letter, send a text, make a call, or even take the person out to dinner with the hope that the emotion of the breakup might be kept to a minimum. What if your meal choices are causing your body to be fatigued? You may want to break up with those bad eating habits, but you have no idea how to start. You may not know why you want to break up, but you know that you are fatigued to the point you're singing the Boyz2Men song, *"Although we have come to the end of the road."* Perhaps you're feeling or using emotion rather than action.

What are some behaviors that could fatigue a relationship? With food?

A. When you are the giver in the relationship, and you've grown tired of that role.
You are not consistent.

B. Incompatibility
You thought you were eating something healthy and it turns out to be something that works against your DNA.
For example: Raw Kale, cauliflower, Brussel sprouts, broccoli, and cabbage interferes with how my thyroid gland uses iodine. I went years eating those vegetables until one day, I started an eating journal because I could hear my heart rate very loud in my ears and explained it to my doctor.

You have lost trust.

C. Cheating
Your cheat days have turned to your everyday way of eating.

D. Too many differences
You don't know where to start (so many choices/varieties of food).

E. Flaws
One research says eating certain foods can be healthy and another study contradicts this.

F. Lack of satisfaction
You want your food to be tasty, not boring.

G. Ineffective communication

(Side note: Did you know vitamin C will not allow iron to absorb into the bloodstream when taken together?)
What sources of vitamins will come from which foods?

H. Suppressed Emotions

Eat to feel better

I. Lack of Time

Don't have time to plan

J. Undefined roles

All these concerns can fatigue even the most skilled healthy eater.

Name some of your behaviors that could fatigue your relationship with food.

_____

_____

_____

_____

_____

_____

_____

_____

_____

_____

_____

_____

_____

_____

_____

_____

_____

_____

_____

Name some of your eating habits that may cause you to feel fatigued and less effective.

_____

_____

_____

_____

_____

_____

_____

_____

_____

_____

_____

_____

_____

_____

_____

_____

_____

_____

As believers, one of the tools that have been handed to us is God's word. When you want to have a deeper walk, and surrender, you can fast. Just like relationships come down to matters of the heart, so will your relationship with the LORD. Man looks at the outer appearance, but God looks at the heart. If the heart isn't transformed during the fasting period, what did the temple gain?

Legacy is not just about the amount of money, or number of houses and land you will leave your children and their children. Legacy serves a greater purpose. You can be a living legacy of a healthy lifestyle.

Language isn't translated; to feel full or to fill satisfied. Some food and ingredients I can't even pronounce.

Countries around the world still practice eating with a purpose. Grandmother used to say, "*Eat your carrots because it's good for your eyes. Eat your spinach because it will make you stronger.*" Let's get back to these types of conversations, rather than conversation urging *eat what you want and when it shows up in your health or your waistline, call a doctor to get it off or take it out.*

Test Your Endurance. Do Those Things You Dare Not Do

Being part of a military family as a child and then marrying a man in the military as an adult, I'm accustomed to moving often. Change is not a matter of *if*, but *when*. Living this type of lifestyle, I came to accept that faith is the extension of doing something, saying something, or giving something.

After living in Okinawa, Japan for less than a month, I decided to be more adventurous and step outside of my comfort zone. I spoke to my husband about being a part of what's called the Dragon Boat Team. My husband signed me up to be on the Army Spouse Dragon Boat Team. He came home one day and said, "Mama, I signed you up for the team. All you have to do is rent a paddle from the gym and show up at Okuma Beach for practice twice a week, for two hours." I thought, *that sounds easy enough*. I got up the next day to go rent my paddle. I was ready to go to the first practice. I put on my designer sweatsuit with matching sneakers. I wore a cap with the word *Okinawa* stitched on the front. I was still learning how to navigate through the city, not to mention driving on the opposite side of the road. Needless to say, I managed to get to Okuma Beach safely.

As I approached the dock area; I didn't see the boat. I thought I was either early or my husband had the wrong time. I proceeded to drive down the rocky dirt road. I saw other women who appeared to be American, gathering near the ocean. I drove into the allotted parking space. Glancing out at the water I noticed a few women were in the water and others were walking towards the water. I was confused because I still did not see a boat. However, as I sat in my car with the car still running, I saw a platform raft floating in the water. One by one, some of the women hopped onto the raft. Each woman turned to help the other woman get on the raft. I quickly realized the *raft* was the actual *boat*. Well, by now it's time for me to get a paddle and join them. I was nervous about this adventure, but excited about being on the team. At the paddle rental booth, one of the employees told me the Dragon Boat event was one of the highlights on the island. It was such a huge event that it was a school holiday. Service members were given a family day pass to attend or participate, plus bragging rights for each military branch who won.

I started walking towards the water with my paddle in hand,

dressed in my cute sweatsuit, matching hat, and sneakers. I definitely had a strut about me that said I was confident. As I got closer to getting into the water, my bold strut turned into a tiptoe. I'm thinking out loud, "How am I going to get to that raft?" I couldn't figure how I was going to get to the raft without getting my entire body wet. *Take off your sweatsuit. What about my feet? That water looks so green. No telling what's at the bottom of the ocean,* I thought. Did I fail to mention, I really don't care much for the beach and can only swim well enough to hopefully save myself? In the meantime, several other women passed me going into the water. One of them stopped to say, "Are you here for the Army Spouse's Dragon Boat practice?" I answered with great confidence, "Yes, I am. She said, "Great. Come on, practice is about to start."

I noticed two women wearing bikini tops with swimming shorts and another one had on a scuba diving suit. There I was, looking like I was either going for a jog or going to teach a Zumba class. Either way, I was not prepared for what was to come. I quickly removed my jacket, shoes, and socks. I could not take off anything else without exposing my girly goodies. I quickly put my shoes back on because I didn't want to touch whatever might be in the ocean water. Immediately, with each step into the water, my sneakers became infused with water. That did not stop me. With paddle over my head and my clothes getting soaked, I began to feel water collect into my bra space! I realized I could no longer walk out to get onto the raft. I felt like I was walking

19

a plank. I was going to drown if I didn't stop walking and start swimming. Before I made the connection that walking was not an option, with the next step I took, I went under, taking in a mouthful of ocean seaweed water. I know I said earlier that I could swim well enough to save my life. Well, the truth is the last time I involuntarily tested that theory was about 17 years ago when I almost drowned in the deep end of a friend's pool!

Back to me getting nature's nutrients from the ocean; All at once, I felt hands grabbing me by my shirt, pulling me out of the water, and onto the raft. When I looked up, I saw one woman holding my paddle, another one had my designer shades and pink cap, and the third one asked if I was okay and if I knew how to swim. I shook my head. All the confidence I had on shore was washed away in the bottom of the ocean! I could do nothing but laugh. The women laughed too after I assured them I was okay.

The actual practice wasn't as eventful as my start. When practice came to an end and it was time for us to get off the raft, the coach offered to help me. You see, the raft had drifted farther out into the ocean. I looked around and saw one woman after another, jump off the raft and into the water, making their way back to shore. There were two other teammates who needed help to get back, but I was determined not to be one of those women who needed help. I graciously declined the coach's offer. Coach insisted that I leave my paddle and she would bring it over. I thought back to how I was taught to swim. *Hold your breath, keep*

your legs and arms moving, and you will get to where you're going.
I jumped off the raft into that seaweed water and began
dog paddling until I felt my feet hit the sand. The coach
was behind me the entire time with my paddle. When she
exited the water, she handed me my paddle and with a hint
of hesitation, she asked, "Will we see you Thursday?" My
confidence returned on dry land and I replied, "You sure
will."

I got my dry sweat jacket and socks off the dock and with
my feet squishing and squeaking with every step, I made it
back to my car. I was proud of myself for not giving up. I
suddenly remembered that I didn't bring a towel or a change
of clothes. I got into the car on the driver's side, glad I left
the keys under the seat or else they might be floating
somewhere in the ocean. I started laughing loud and hard. I
was sitting in a puddle of water from my ocean experience.
I rolled down my window in hopes that my clothes would
quickly dry from the 110 degree heat. Next, I turned on the
radio. I kid you not, the song playing on the radio was *I
wish they all could be California girls* . I began to laugh again.
Not only because I'm a southern girl who was trying to act
like I was a California girl, but because of what I had just
experienced. How timely. As I'm driving along, my clothes
and hair started to dry. My hair had begun its
transformation from straight to natural. At this point, it had
been about two years since my last hair relaxer. My cute
pink hat with the words *Okinawa* began rising on top of my

21

head. Oh, LAWD! By the time I made it home, my hat was sitting on a mountain of all-natural hair!

My husband and daughter were sitting in the family room when I walked into the house. My husband spoke first. He asked me how practice went, followed by my daughter. My daughter looked up, spoke to me, and then wanted to know what had happened to my hair, to my clothes, and why were my sneakers squeaking. I couldn't answer either of them. All I could do was start laughing again. All the way to the bathroom, I kept thinking about what had happened. *I am so glad I know how to swim just like I was a child. Well enough to save my life.*

I shared this story with you because I want you to know or be reminded that it is okay. After all, 40's is the new 20's, 50's and 60's is the new 30's. I understand there are times when we want to go back and be childlike, but remember to make adult decisions to save your life. I encourage you to give your child a safety net of healthy eating and exercise that can allow them to live well into the seasoned and wise 90's.

Side note: I discovered two weeks later, at the ripe old age of 47, I was pregnant with our "Okinawa Surprise." I still completed the season and rowed with the team! I guess the seaweed water was just the nutrient my body needed to withstand the physical demands of gaining life.

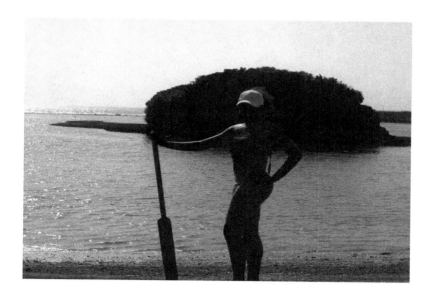

Instead Of Raising Children, RAISE EXPECTATIONS

Train up a child in the way he should go; and when he is old, he will not depart from it. Proverbs 22:6 KJV

I have heard many people say, "We do not have a book on how to raise a child." To some degree that statement has some truth to it. I challenge you to stop raising children and raise expectations.

Early development of children is driven by parents (caregivers). It is like having a GPS to tell you how to get home. Whether you realize it or not, children watch your relationship with food. The relationship is passed on to your grandchildren and their grandchildren. This nutritional journey doesn't have to be complicated.

Many years ago, driving home from work, my oldest daughter who was around two and a half, maybe three at the time, was in the back seat in her car seat. "Mommy, we're almost home. Our house is over there," she said, pointing. We were at least two blocks from home. I asked her how she knew we were almost home. She said, "Because the roof is red." Sure, enough the house on the corner, entering our subdivision, had a red roof. The remaining roofs were black. What I did not take into account was that I had driven the same route for at least a year, and although she did not know how to drive or understand directions, she knew her shapes, colors and could count to twenty (20). This speaks to how children gather information from their parents (caregivers), as well as their environment. Furthermore, it is driven home with the use of physical movement and how you, as a parent (caregiver), live your daily lives. The message should be daily and consistent. At some point, the child(ren) will begin to make decisions on their own.

According to a new study from The University of Washington, by age 5, kids develop important personality traits. Hint: It has to do with confidence. By the time your child heads off to school—kindergarten even—their self-esteem might already be fully developed and like that of an adult. What if parents started using a GPS approach to parenting? Perhaps having insight to recognize you are not raising children, but raising expectations in our adults. Parents start with them at an early age, taking your adults to work at home. Remember to give them a 90-day probation with an "O, I see day" to help them with some challenges of the orientation. Learning starts at ground zero in the home. I believe it would make a positive difference if each household came up with their own written orientation, covenant, and instruction booklet like one would get when starting a new job. Set your legacies (children) up for success: 1) Walk them through each area of the house, 2) Show them how to start and complete a task. Some parents feel like their children have been watching them, (they have), so the children should know what to do around the house. That may be true, but sometimes our actions aren't consistent with our words. The feedback I have heard from some parents prior to covid-19 and virtual learning is some parents feel they do not need to *micromanage* their children. That is not what I am suggesting.

However, what I *am* saying is parents, we should teach our legacies to C.A.R.E (Community Accountability Responsibility for Each other). Sometimes this can be accomplished by doing those things you or the children may not necessarily care about. This can help build a concern to care about other people even when you don't have to. As a suggestion, you could use a booklet like the example on the following pages.

MEDICAL CLINIC (KNOWN AS THE KITCHEN)

Wash hands upon entering this clinic.

The refrigerator is your medicine cabinet. It stores the food you need to nourish your body. The pantry is the second medicine cabinet. The pantry stores dried foods and seasonings that provide taste for your food.

Food is nourishment for the body; it is to be used for fuel to maintain your level of energy during activities of daily living.

I. Be considerate of everyone in the household when you're in the clinic.
A. A clean kitchen is not your opportunity to leave it unclean.
   I. Clean up after yourself.

B. There is a time and place.

   I. Breakfast
   2. Lunch
   3. Dinner
   4. Snacks (be considerate of others who want snacks as well)

ORDER OF MEDICAL CLINIC

Appliances, counter tops, floor, and cabinets are not cleaned through osmosis.

RANGE (OVEN) AND STOVE TOP

Once you have acquired the skill set to safely operate the oven, make sure you clean up any spills whether you spilled it or not.

COUNTER TOPS

Are to remain:

1. Free of clutter, cups, plates, etc.
2. Clean them. A clean surface is NOT your opportunity to make it unclean for anyone else in the household to clean up behind you.

FLOOR

Floor should be debris free. If you spill something on the floor, clean it up right then and there.

1. Use a mop, damp paper towels or napkins, or anything disposable to clean the spill.
2. Wear slippers, socks, or bare feet on all floor areas in the house.
3. Clean up spills and mess immediately.

CONTINUING ORDER OF THE MEDICAL CLINIC SINK AND GARBAGE DISPOSAL

Once you have acquired the skill set of washing dishes:

1. Wash dishes immediately after each meal or snack.
2. No dishes are to be left in the sink during the day.
3. Use paper products (cups, utensils, plates), unless instructed to use regular cups, utensils, and plates.
4. Wiping down counter tops, range, refrigerator, cabinets, dishwasher, sweeping, and/or mopping is part of doing the dishes.

GARBAGE DISPOSAL

1. Keep strainer over garbage disposal, and empty any extra food or debris that might have gotten into it.
2. Refrain from using the garbage disposal.

DISHWASHER

Once you have acquired the skill set on how to use the dishwasher, do not turn it on.

1. It is to be used to store and wash dishes.
2. Dishes are to be cleared out of the dishwasher the next morning.
3. Wipe down inside of dishwasher after clearing

and putting away the dishes.

TRASH

1. Is to be taken out daily (prior to going to bed).
2. Sanitation service usually picks up trash on scheduled days of the week, depending on the weather. Take trash can to curb the night before pickup or by 6:30 am the morning of pickup.

For some of you, the above may appear to be over the top; yet you are continuously asking young people to clean up behind themselves. Others of you may feel this goes without saying. Most kids rise to the occasion when expectations are discussed along with times and dates. This way, details can be understood and agreed upon.

RESTORATION ROOM (KNOWN AS THE BEDROOM)

Getting enough quality **sleep** at the right time can help protect your mental health, physical health, quality of life, and safety.

A good night's sleep starts in the morning.

"If you want to change the world,
start off by making your bed."
Admiral William McRaven

1. Rise
2. Make your bed
3. 5-10 minutes meditation/prayer
4. Get dressed for the day
5. Breakfast
6. Play/Activities/Social
   A. Go to recreation room or outside
7. Get in 1-2 hours of physical exercise daily (leisure physical activity is important)
8. Exercise your brain 1-2 hours daily

Sleep plays a vital role in good health and
well-being throughout your life. Your
mental strength is counting on you to get
the appropriate amount of sleep.

SLEEP HYGIENE

1. To increase the chances of resting well, your bed is to be used for sleeping at night.
2. You may decide to read prior to going to bed.
   A. If you cannot sleep, step out of your bed and sit in a chair in your room. Allow your mind to be quiet.
   B. If it has been longer than 30 minutes, get out of bed. Go sit in a quiet place.
   C. Write down those things that are on your mind.
   - If you must nap during the day, a rule of thumb is to nap for no more than 10-20

minutes

ORAL HYGIENE

Brushing your teeth is an important step in growing up
healthy.

Oral hygiene can be an important indicator in spotlighting
your inside health either by the way your teeth and gums
look or by the odor of your breath. What you eat will show
up on your teeth. The bacteria will get on your tongue.
The following suggestions may be a no-brainer for some
of you. However, there are children and adults who do not
know how the quality of their lives can change by being
consistent with their oral hygiene and making regular
visits to a dentist at least two times a year.

Just like washing dishes, the detail is not limited to
washing dishes only; you should clean the whole
kitchen. When it comes to oral hygiene, brushing your
teeth is not just brushing your teeth. You should:

1. Brush your teeth

    A. Three times a day

- Morning
- Noon
- Night

2. Instrument or tools to use

A. Electric toothbrush
B. Water pick
C. Dental floss

- Three times a day
- In between snacks and meals

D. Tongue scraper
E. Rinse

3. Last step: Drink eight (8) ounces of water after you are finished (morning and noon).

4. Change your toothbrush or toothbrush head at least four (4) times a year, especially during cold and flu season.

CONFERENCE ROOM (DINING ROOM)

1. Team building/meeting to come to a clear understanding and to follow up on any unresolved issue(s)
2. Set a weekly family/team check in time.
3. Use an agenda or notebook to write down issues you would like to discuss at the meeting.
4. The meeting should last about one (1) hour.
5. Presentations should not be longer than 10 minutes.
6. All voices will be heard.
7. Be respectful of others and their opinions.
8. Solutions don't always happen overnight.

ADMINISTRATION ROOM
(HOME OFFICE)

Area designated for academic learning PRAYER/
READING

ROOM
(PRAYER CLOSET)

This house is built on prayer. Gain knowledge, discipleship, and a relationship with our Lord and Savior.

1. Anytime prayer/devotion/meditation
2. Room reserved for peace
3. Gain a deeper understanding of
   A. Your self-worth
   B. That you matter
   C. Your purpose
      ○ Purpose can be determined on any given day.

COMPUTER

We are in an era of technology. Having this tool can be very instrumental in remaining current with how the world communicates today. If we aren't careful with our young minds; it can be harmful

Growing up, my parents would tell us not allow anyone to come into the house, once they were gone to run errands and we could not go outside the home until they returned.

These days our children are online or engaging in social media without physical parental guidance (not the kind that is placed on the devices); this is just like letting someone into your home, who you do not know.

Dare to Parent, provide limitation and reinforce the expectations.

To use the computer there must be:

1. An agreement about the usage prior to getting on the computer.
2. Skill set (for the younger kids in the house).
   A. When a child starts learning how to use the computer, they need a lesson from the parent(s) about proper usage.

CHANGE STARTS IN YOUR MIND. FOLLOW IT WITH YOUR ACTIONS, LOVE, PEACE, AND KINDNESS

Family Fun Chore

BREAK ACTIVITIES

SOCK BANDIT ACTIVITY

First step: Put on a pair of socks (hint: knee high socks) leave loose in the toe area.

Second step: Place your feet on the floor (either in a circle to start or across from family members).

Third step: Count 1-2-3 and say the word: (Say your family name).

Fourth step: using your feet only, try to take off the socks of your family member(s).

1. You are in a crab walk position.
2. You cannot stand up.
3. You cannot tuck your feet underneath anything.

4. Your feet must remain on the floor at all times.

5. You cannot use your hands.

CLEAN YOUR ROOM ACTIVITY

1. Use soft, tossable object (foam balls, bean bags, and crumpled paper) per 4 family members.
2. Designate a play area.
3. Get family teams, one on each side.
4. Place an even amount of objects on each side.
5. When you give the *start* cue, have each family team member pick-up and throw from their side to the other side.

BALLOON VOLLEY BALL ACTIVITY

1. Use one balloon (or as many balloons as you like) and make a partition to play a game of volleyball.
2. Stand, kneel, or sit.
3. You can make up your own rules.
4. Have fun and keep moving, taking a break from the chores.

Using Our Minutes

"And the house which I build is great: for great is our God above all gods." 2 *Chronicles* 2:5 *KJV*

What if the Bible was like our cell phones?

What if you carried your Bible with you each day and checked it throughout the day for messages. You go over your *data plan* each month. You tweet, Instagram, Facebook and text about it daily. When you leave home, you turn around, go back and get it. You feel insecure without it. You make sure your children carry it to school and have it with them at night. When you can't sleep, you check it for messages.

DNA is coded by strands that match us to other people. There are brackets that fit perfectly giving scientists the ability to match children with parents and grandparents as well as ancestors from generations past. If you know your past, this can be a template for what your health walk might look like.

In 2018, I was watching the USA Women's Ice Hockey team play for the gold medal against Canada. At some point during the game, I fell asleep and missed the ending of the game. I remember the score being 2-1 at the top of the third period. It looked like the USA would have to settle for another silver medal.

The next morning, I tried to avoid hearing the results because I wanted to re-watch it later. I made it the entire day and did not hear about who had won! Prior to going to bed, I was reading a bedtime story to my daughter and catching up on her day. We finished reading the book and I tucked her in and said my usual *goodnight* and *I love you*. She said, "I love you too" and then she said, "Mommy, you know who probably is having a hard time sleeping tonight?" I said, "No, who?" She said, "The winners, the USA Women's Hockey team!"

I walked to the family room and turned on the game. The commentator announced the USA Women's Ice Hockey team had not won a gold medal since 1998. I watched the re-televised broadcast. I was watching the game as if I did not already know the outcome. I was screaming and yelling at the ladies like I was going to change their movements. I finally saw the end result of the shootout shot that secured the gold medal.

This reminds me how we can forget and doubt God's promises. God's word says He made us in His own image. God has provided instructions about His nutritional laws. Start today by changing your nutritional habits. You have the information about your DNA. Just like a house you purchased that was built 90 years ago, you can decide to rebuild and restore it. You can change the home, and add more rooms essential for your family to live in now. You do not have to agree with the history of your DNA. Just like the shootout in the hockey game that changed from the USA team possibly getting the silver medal to them securing the gold medal, you can make the change just as quickly. Read your Bible daily. Pick it up to gain knowledge and receive messages. Build generations of believers and disciples who are willing to house the "Great I Am."

You may work 9-10 hours outside of your home. During the waking hours some of you will have three meals a day and snacks in between. Plan when you are going to eat your meals. Have an idea of what you want to eat. People can get caught in a trap when they only eat what's available. For example, if asked to go out to lunch or if there is a celebration in the office they will go with what the crowd is eating.

How do you decide what to eat? Plan what you are going to eat. Do not let the environment influence your decision. My sister likes the quote, "If you don't stand for something, you will fall for anything."

Try to eat the healthiest meals. Limit to eating at home
1. You don't have to eat unhealthy often.
2. You can plan when you are going to do it.
3. You will get what satisfies your taste buds.

Do you attend social functions and eat and drink any and everything available, and then when you leave you reflect on your evening and think, *what a great time I had!* Some parts of the evening might remind you of times when you were in your 20's when you could eat anything you wanted. Fast forward, the next morning after overeating, you are quickly reminded that you cannot eat and drink like that any longer because you are not in your 20's. You're 40!

Chapter 5: 2-3

BASEBALL

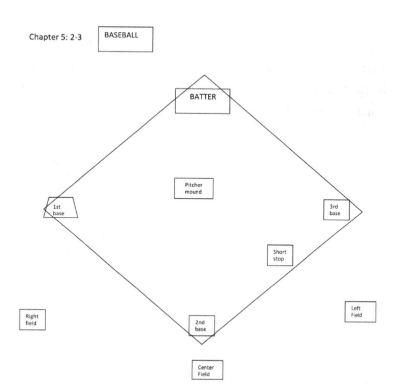

Like the game of baseball, each person on the team has a certain position to play. The ball represents God's word. Write the word on a strip of paper, ball it up, and put the word into play. Hit the ball!

A.	Deuteronomy 8	___(2) Oh Lord, you have searched me! You know when I sit down and when I rise; You discern my thoughts from afar (3)You search out of my path and my lying down and are acquainted with my ways.
B.	Psalm 139: 1-3	___(5) The apostles said to the Lord increase our faith! (6) And the Lord said, If you had faith like a grain of mustard seed. You could say to this mulberry tree; Be uprooted and planted in the sea; and it would obey you.
C.	Luke 17: 5-6	___(8) A land of wheat, and barley and vines, a fig tree and pomegranates; a land of olive oil and honey.
D.	John 6:35	___(22) A joyful heart is good medicine, but a crushed spirit dries up the bones.
E.	Proverbs 17:22	_(35) Jesus said to them. " I am the bread of life; whoever comes to me shall not hunger, and whoever believes in me shall never thirst.
F.	1 Corinthians 10:31	_(2) Beloved, I pray that all may go well with you and that you may be in good health, as it goes well with your soul.
G.	3 John 1:2	___(31) So, whether you eat or drink, or whatever you do, do all to the glory of God.

Sitting Is The New Smoking

Oxygen is the life supporting component of the air we breathe which makes our lives breathable. With COVID-19 (coronavirus), there is a lot spoken about oxygen and how those that are at high risk have a need for optimal levels of oxygen. The air we breathe could become very harmful to us. Once that message was received people worldwide began to order respiratory and oxygen machines. During the coronavirus it has been suggested, when in public, to wear a face covering.

The USDA suggests we eat more vegetables, fruits, whole grains, fat free or 1% milk, and dairy products. These foods have the nutrients needed for optimal health, including potassium, calcium, vitamins D and E, and fiber. The food pyramid can be the template for your meals. As parents, one of our greatest responsibilities to our children is to feed them. We are also accountable for what we feed them. One thing about legacy is that you will be one of the creators at some point in your life. What you make of this is what can be passed down to generations to come. This will be your own creation. I pass no judgment; I understand all too well that resources for some are a lot more challenging than for others. Nevertheless, we can all make a choice to be more active and do less sitting around. Even when watching television, you can play what I call *the commercial game*. During each commercial do something physical. You can even put the remote out of reach so you have to walk to get it. One of the exercises I do during commercials is couch sit-ups. The options are endless.

According to the CDC, the life expectancy of a smoker is at least 10 years shorter than non-smokers. However, sitting too much can increase your risk for poor health outcomes. The strongest risk of sitting too much is diabetes. Sitting too much doubles the risk, so get to moving, and keep moving as often and as much as possible.

I am a former physical education teacher, basketball, and track and field coach for 25 plus years. The amount of time students spend in physical education class has declined significantly. However, over time, enrollment in paying programs has increased in order to make up for these programs not being available in a growing number of schools. The expectation and standards are different for those who wish to pursue extracurricular activities. This may be known as *you get a trophy era*. I once heard someone say that it takes a village to raise a child. Once the curriculum for physical education changed, half the village was sidelined.

Looking at the history of our country, as it relates to fitness and health in schools, many U.S. presidents have been instrumental in working towards a solution. On the other hand, they have fallen short of solving the obesity crisis in adults and children.

According to U.S. Department of Health & Human Services (hhs.gov), United States of America Presidents have tried with some success and some failures to get children moving and encourage adults to live a healthier lifestyle. As of 2018, most efforts were slowing down or nonexistent.

ADMINISTRATION: 1953-1961
DWIGHT D. EISENHOWER

As a military man, President Dwight D. Eisenhower was probably already sensitive to the issue of physical fitness. Military officers grumbled about the condition of draftees during World War and the Korean War. Concern about fitness peaked in the mid-1950s with publication of an international study that found American children far less fit than children in other countries. In response, President Eisenhower established the President's Council on Youth Fitness with Executive Order 10673, issued July 16, 1956.

ADMINISTRATION: 1961-1963
JOHN F. KENNEDY

In the end, another crucial factor that prevented the President's Council from reaching its full potential is the inattentiveness of the president. Having established the council, Eisenhower rarely spoke on the subject of fitness. Neither did he appear at any of its annual conferences. John F. Kennedy's approach to the problem of fitness would be very different.

ADMINISTRATION: 1963-1969
LYNDON B JOHNSON

The Presidential Physical Fitness Award is the highest award given for performance on the AAHPER (American Association for Health, Physical Education and Recreation) Youth Fitness Test. Established by President Lyndon B. Johnson in 1966, this award honors students who demonstrate exceptional physical achievement.

In 1966, Presidential Youth Fitness Program was established to help address the New York State Journal of Medicine reported 4,400 students between the ages 6 and 16 in the public system across the United States.

ADMINISTRATION: 1969-1974
RICHARD M NIXON

Under the Nixon administration, the Council expands the

Presidential Physical Fitness Awards to include recreation departments and groups, such as boys' and girls' clubs. In 1970, special advisors are developed to stimulate the development of physical fitness programs for employees. It enhanced public relation activities and instigated the possibility of private support for Council projects.

ADMINISTRATION: 1974-1977
GERALD R. FORD

The Executive Order is amended with two additional objectives in 1976. The first additional objective is to *charge* the Council with informing the general public of the importance of exercise. The second objective is to assist businesses and industries with establishing sound physical fitness programs.

In 1975, the third National Youth Fitness Survey takes place. The results do not show as much improvement as the survey in 1965.

ADMINISTRATION: 1977-1981
JAMES E. CARTER

During President Carter's tenure, Council membership expands to 15 members. In 1979, physical fitness and exercise become one of 15 priority areas in a national health promotion/disease prevention initiative with the Council as the lead agency.

In addition to Congress passing the Amateur Sports Act of 1978, reorganizing the United States Olympic Committee, President Carter speaks at first National Conference on Physical Fitness.

ADMINISTRATION: 1981-1989
RONALD W. REAGAN

In 1983, the White House Symposium on Physical Fitness and Sports Medicine established. May proclaimed National Physical Fitness and Sports Month.

In 1984, National Conference on Youth Fitness and six regional public hearings on physical fitness and physical education takes place. The first National Women's Leadership Conference on Fitness takes place with First Lady Nancy Reagan as Honorary Chair.

In 1987, the Amateur Athletic Union awarded contract to administer today's President's Challenge.

In the public health arena, the Council reports on the 1990 Objectives in the exercise and fitness priority area.

ADMINISTRATION: 1989-1993
GEORGE W. BUSH

In 1989, the Council is named the lead agency on physical activity and fitness priority area of Healthy People 2000, with CDC as the science advisor.

In 1990, the National Conference on Military Fitness takes place to review important physical fitness issues facing service members.

In 1991, the Participant Physical Fitness Award is added. The Presidential Sports Award recognizes the first family that earns the Family Fitness Award.

Administration: 1993-2001
William J. Clinton

1997, Fit Start is added to the Presidential Sports and Health Fitness Awards. Material made available in Spanish.

In cooperation with the National Archive and Records Administration, the Council sponsors *Flexing the Nation's Muscle: President's, Physical Fitness and Sports in the American Century*, a traveling exhibit featuring twentieth century presidents and their participation in activity and fitness. Sponsored by Sporting Goods Manufacturers Association (SGMA) and International Health, Racquet and Sportsclub Association (IHRSA), the Council partnered with the Advertising Council to develop a 3-year ad campaign focusing on youth fitness, "Get Off It!" and "Get Up, Get Out."

The Council and CDC are named co-leads for the physical activity and fitness goals of *Healthy People 2010* and physical activity is named one of 10 *Leading Health Indicators*. President Clinton issues Executive Memorandum directing Secretaries of HHS and Education to identify strategies to improve the nation's youth fitness. In November 2000, a report is presented to the White House, *Promoting Better Health for Young People through Physical Activity and Sports.*

ADMINISTRATION: 2001-2009
GEORGE W. BUSH JR.

For the 2001-02 school year, the President's Challenge expands to three areas and the Presidential Active Lifestyle Award is made available for children and youth. On June 16, 2004, Healthier US Fitness Festival is held on the National Mall with the Congressional Fitness Caucus. A year later, on May 2, 2005, the second Healthier US Fitness Festival is held on the National Mall to observe National Physical Fitness and Sports Month.

The third Healthier US Fitness Challenge is held at RFK Stadium in Washington, DC to celebrate National Physical Fitness and Sports Month on May 6, 2006. In fall 2007, the second Healthier Feds Physical Activity Challenge is held. The expanded program included all three branches of government and independent agencies. Approximately 40,000 federal workers, contractors, and their family members register.

On May 14, 2008, the Council launched the new national Adult Fitness Test at an event held at a local gym in

Washington, DC with the International Health, Racquet and Sportsclub Association.

On October 7, 2008, HHS releases the first Physical Activity Guidelines for Americans. The launch was followed by a partnership forum run by the Council and the Office of Disease Prevention and Health Promotion, which served as the leading offices in the development of the Guidelines.

ADMINISTRATION: 2009-2017
BARACK H. OBAMA

June 23, 2010, White House announces new Presidential Executive Order changing the Council's name to the President's Council on Fitness, Sports and Nutrition, expands the mission of the Council to include nutrition, and increases the number of Council members from 20 to 25.

September 14, 2010, First Lady Michelle Obama and HHS Secretary Kathleen Sebellus announce the Million PALA Challenge to get one million Americans to complete the Presidential Active Lifestyle Award (PALA). Between Sept 2010 and Sept 2011 1.7 million Americans earned their PALA.

September 10, 2012, President's Council launches the Presidential Youth Fitness Program (PYFP), a comprehensive school-based program that employs the latest science and promotes health and physical activity for America's youth, phasing out and replacing the Youth Fitness Test that dates back to 1966.

February 2013, President's Council and First Lady Michelle Obama launch Let's Move! Active Schools, a solution to ensure 60 minutes of physical activity every day is the norm in schools across America.

March 2013, Physical Activity Guidelines for Americans Midcourse Report: Strategies to increase Physical Activity Among Youth, is released by the Department of Health and Human Services as a five-year follow up to the 2008 Physical Activity Guidelines for Americans.

In January 2017, the Council's Presidential Champions program is incorporated into the U.S. Department of Agriculture's Super Tracker Food and Nutrition Tracking Tool.

ADMINISTRATION: 2017-PRESENT
DONALD J. TRUMP

June 30, 2018, the Presidential Champions program is discontinued. Presidential Champions was an online only program that was integrated into USDA's Super Tracker in January 2017. Therefore, with the discontinuation of Super Tracker, the President's Council on Sports, Fitness & Nutrition discontinued the Presidential Champions program.

June 10, 2019, the President's Council on Sports, Fitness & Nutrition is merged with the Office of Disease Prevention and Health Promotion (ODPHP). The merging of PCSFN and ODPHP, which was announced April 10, 2019, is part of a new structure for the Office of the Assistant Secretary for Health (OASH).

June 21, 2019, the Office of the Assistant Secretary for Health (OASH) announces its intent to reinstate the President's Council on Sports, Fitness & Nutrition Science Board.

Do It For The Vine

I am the Vine, ye are the branches, he who abides in Me and I in him, the same bringeth forth much fruit, for without Me, Ye can do nothing. John 15:5 KJV

In high school, I played basketball and I was on the intramural team in college. I was also a conditioning coach at the collegiate level for the girls' basketball team. In high school, my position was the number one guard and small forward. In the game of basketball, there are five team members from each team on the court at the same time. The objective of the game is to score more points than your opponent before the allotted time runs out on the clock. Each position contributes to the process of how the team operates. Before the operation of the position or game is played or a point scored, the team started with a plan (the vine).

If I look at the character of our team like the parts of a tree,

I would assign each team member the following; the coach equals the *soil*, assistant coach equals the *roots*, managers, personal trainers, maintenance personal who keep the locker rooms and gym clean, towel person, team physician, and parents equal the *tree, and* the team members are the *branches*.

Before basketball season started, whenever my coach saw me in the hall he would say, "Spider" (a nick name that grew on me), "are you ready for the season?" My response would often be "Yes, Coach." What got get me is Coach required me to run on the cross-country team so I would be in condition by the time basketball season rolled around. He didn't do that just to me; he did it with everybody on the team. Each one of us had to be involved in a school activity, mainly a sport activity. Coach would make sure we were basketball ready with conditioning drills or strongly suggesting we have physical education as one of our class electives. At the start of basketball season, we did not go directly to the X's and O's of our offense and defense. We started with conditioning. I couldn't believe the amount of conditioning we did at the start and end of each practice. Coach already knew we had been involved in other sports and we would come into the season well-conditioned and ready to go. Once I became a coach, I understood all too well why being in basketball shape is different than being in cross- country or track shape. For the first two weeks of practice, no basketball was handed out other than to shoot free throws and to weed out potential teammates. Coach would have us doing drills called *suicide* (coaches weren't as sensitive to society's feelings back then) to name a drill that name. The drill started with us standing behind the backboard on the black line. We would run as fast as we could to reach and touch each horizontal line, and return to the start. We continued the suicide drill until we touched the last line on the opposite end of the court and then we sprinted back to the starting black line.

Even if you, as an individual, finished the drill within the allotted time, if the rest of the team did not make it within a certain time frame, we had to do it again and again either until we made the time together or the coach got tired. That was one of many drills we did before and after practice. Each drill incorporated teamwork. Whether we failed or succeeded it was together. Once the season was in full bloom, we were ready for the Xs and Os of our game plan (the vine). Prior to taking the court, our coach or another teammate would lead us in the Lord's Prayer.

Our Father, who art in heaven, hallowed be thy name; thy kingdom come; thy will be done; on earth as it is in heaven. Give us this day our daily bread. And forgive us our trespasses, as we forgive those who trespass against us. And lead us not into temptation; but deliver us from evil. For thine is the kingdom, the power and the glory, for ever and ever. Amen.

As a fourteen-year-old girl, I didn't understand why we said that prayer. However, after playing the game of basketball there was a lot of forgiveness that had to happen. For instance, I had to forgive my coach for cursing out the referee. I had to forgive myself for going after the ball and sitting on my opponent's back in order to gain possession of the ball, even after the whistle had blown and the play was over....

GAME TIME! Coaches (the soil and the tree) had done their parts. It's time for the team to produce (the branches) the fruits of our labor. We won many of our games because every teammate (branches) operated at an optimal level (produced much fruit), mainly by sticking to the plan (the vine). Other nights, we fell apart at the root because we didn't come together as a team. Some teammates had their own agendas, others started going against the game plan (the vine). Nothing came together. That's when we experienced most of our losses.

In high school, I earned numerous basketball awards, including MVP, All District, All Regional, and Honorable Mention. Valuable lessons and foundations were set so I would know how to transfer those basketball drills into tangible life skills. When I went to college, I was awarded a track scholarship but I still used my coach's principle of being in condition. I joined our intramural basketball team. My college teammates were some of the same opponents I played against in high school. My branch attached to theirs. They were some terrific basketball players and even better friends.

As I grew from high school basketball to intramural

basketball in college, the levels were certainly different, but what remained the same was the game. What changed was we didn't have someone telling us to get ready for the season. One of our teammate brothers agreed to coach us, but it wasn't the same as our high school coaches (soil). We had to become the roots, the tree, and the branches. Most of us drew from our earlier days of basketball so it turned out to be a good fit. We won all of our intramural games, except during the championship when we got beat by women who played volleyball for the University. What I didn't know then that I know now, is the volleyball team was still connected to the vine (plan). They had a volleyball coach (the soil), the other support staff (the tree), and they were teammates (branches) who still did drills and team building exercises. We had the love for the game, we were talented athletes, and we wanted to play together, but we didn't attend to the soil. Therefore, we did not have a plan (the vine).

Oprah Winfrey said, "Use your life as a classroom." When I started coaching, I attempted to do just that. I was a college conditioning coach. I carried a lot of what I knew from my years as an athlete from my degree(s) and life experiences. At this coaching level, my understanding of the game of basketball evolved from my childhood years through young adulthood. In my childhood years, my coach fed me with the knowledge he had. He nurtured me by guiding me through the process of becoming a basketball player. He provided me with a game plan of what to do, even when I wasn't playing basketball, by encouraging me to participate in other conditions that would support me during basketball. I didn't mention earlier when I ran cross country, I hated it! I had such a mediocre attitude during cross-country season, something I had apologized for later when I was teaching at my old high school and my cross-country coach was still the biology teacher there. Although we won three or four State championships, I didn't recognize that my mental attitude was being shaped. I had a mental toughness that would serve me well much later in life. I took the same principles my coach provided and applied them to my life. 1. Use other resources to develop the whole person (associate with like-minded people). 2. Be game ready even in the off season (write down your plan). 3. The richness of your soil can determine how strong and how much fruit your tree will produce on and off the court (identify your needs). 4. When you're going down the unplanned path, it's okay to hit the reset button. 5. Be a team player in most situations. Be willing to help others get what they want or need out of life (be selfless).

The breakout of COVID-19 around the world in 2020 caused many of us to pause and assess what's really important in our lives. There will not be any brackets for your college basketball teams. What if we were able to choose which part of our DNA we would take with us to give to our children? Everything is passed down. You do not have to be in agreement. You can choose to live your life healthier. What would you choose to take? Look at the bracket below and decide what you would choose if you had to.

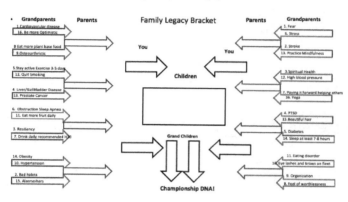

Rewrite Your DNA
(Which Means Do Not Agree)

Example of a family bracket:

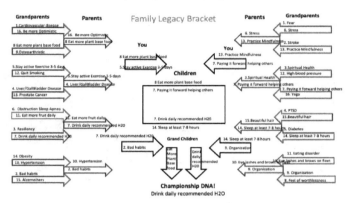

Rewrite Your DNA

(WHICH MEANS YOU DO NOT AGREE)

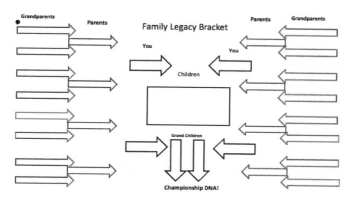

Overpaid Waitress

"Therefore if there is any consolation in Christ, if any comfort of love, if any fellowship of the Spirit, if any affection and mercy, 2 fulfill my joy by being like-minded, having the same love, being of one accord, of one mind. 3 Let nothing be done through selfish ambition or conceit, but in lowliness of mind let each esteem others better than himself. 4 Let each of you look out not only for his own interests, but also for the interests of others. 5 Let this mind be in you which was also in Christ Jesus, 6 who, being in the form of God, did not consider it robbery to be equal with God, 7 but made Himself of no reputation, taking the form of a bondservant, and coming in the likeness of men. 8 And being found in appearance as a man, He humbled Himself and became obedient to the point of death, even the death of the cross." Philippians 2:1-8KJV

I have come to realize that my military up bringing shaped a lot of my decisions. In my early twenties, I became a flight attendant. I enjoyed this job because it allowed me to travel.

As you might already know, extensive training is required to become a flight attendant. There are a lot of situations that could happen in the air. Being prepared to handle those situations is sometimes a matter of life or death. In flight training we had to be mentally in shape as well as emotionally prepared. The first six weeks of training we had CPR training classes, situational training classes, and customer service classes, to name a few. However, we weren't *given* instincts; this training came with experience. One particular flight I especially remember was the time a passenger didn't believe I was qualified to be called a flight attendant. He thought my position was overrated. Most of you are probably familiar with the flight brief the crew gives prior to the plane taking off. On this particular day, I did my routine pre-flight check of the cabin, which consisted of, but not limited to, the following: check lights, seat cushions, fire extinguishers, emergency doors, and oxygen masks. I would touch each seat, overhead compartment, and cockpit while praying over every area of the plane that I could. My prayer was simple but exact. *"Lord, give me patience and discernment to know what to do in an emergency. Allow me to be the voice that will bring calm in the time of a storm. Steady the hands of our pilots and open the ears of our passengers."* Moments after I complete my check, usually the first officer and the captain have completed their flight check as well and soon after we are ready to welcome the passengers aboard. On this particular flight, the captain told me the flight was going to be a bumpy ride, and I may not be able to do the usual in-flight service. With that in mind, I already knew some of the passengers were going to have an issue with that. I know, all too well, I am about to encounter all types of personalities. People from diverse walks of life. I prepare myself by being as pleasant and kind as possible. I made it part of my beginning flight routine to greet each and every passenger as if I was greeting a guest into my home. Passengers board the plane, some with pleasant smiles, others did not look up, and others were preoccupied with their bags and children.

After all passengers were on board and accounted for, the cabin doors were closed and I prepared to start my flight announcement. As I picked up the microphone to speak, a passenger called me over. Since I hadn't started my announcement, I placed the phone back on the receiver and walked to where he was. He asked when I was going to serve. I politely told him I would explain that in a moment. He didn't accept my answer. Rather, he stated, "How difficult is it for you to tell me now?" With a smile on my face, I told him it was not difficult and I would cover that question in my announcement. Just at that time the captain came over the speaker and welcomed the passengers. He explained the flight might experience heavy turbulence so he wanted everyone to keep their seatbelts on whenever the seatbelt sign was on. After the captain was done, I picked up the phone to begin my routine in-flight announcement, part of which was to inform the passengers there would not be an in-flight service due to heavy turbulence. I continued with my normal routine but to recapture the attention of the passengers, when I got to the part about smoking being prohibited in the cabin or lavatory, I threw in a slight joke. I said, "If you feel the need to smoke, please step out onto the wing." Most of the passengers looked up and laughed, but not this one passenger. I thought to myself, *this is going to be an interesting flight.*

I completed my announcement and the captain instructed the attendants to prepare the cabin for takeoff. Just as I was about to sit down, the flight attendant light illuminated. It was the same passenger who wanted to know about the in-flight service. I went to him and he said, "So, you aren't going to serve on this flight?" I told him there would not but I could get him a cup of water before takeoff. He insisted on having something stronger. Again, I politely informed him that I wouldn't be able to serve him and reminded him of what the captain said about turbulence. I followed up with an apology for the inconvenience and asked if there was anything else I could assist him with. After he told me there was nothing I could do, I turned to walk away, he said smugly, "You're nothing but an overpaid waitress!" Of course, I ignored his snide remark and continued to my jump seat.

We took off, and shortly after, turbulence started and continued on and off for the duration of the flight. The seatbelt sign remained illuminated. All passengers were in compliance. The flight attendant light came on again from the same passenger. He asked me for a rum and pop. I said, "Sir, at this time it may appear to be calm, but the storm is just ahead, and we will be experiencing turbulence again." Before turning around and leaving I asked once again if there was anything else I could assist him with. He did not answer me.

The plane began to shake, but before taking my seat I checked on a mom with her baby to see if they were okay. I don't know how, but the baby was sleeping soundly. I went and sat down in my jump seat. The plane lifted in the air and then dropped! All I could think about was what to do in case of an emergency. We finally stopped dropping and the plane just shook. I started praying. I asked God to get us through the storm with all parts of the plane intact, and to steady the hands of the pilots. I prayed over and over. The plane dropped so low I could hear passengers screaming like they were on a rollercoaster ride. Then I heard the baby cry. I got on the microphone and reminded the passengers to remain seated with their seatbelts on. After about five to ten minutes the plane was calm.

Captain got back on the PA and announced he was trying to get around the storm, but it looked like we were going to have to go through it. I could hear passengers talking to each other, concerned. The flight attendant light illuminated. I got on the PA and informed the passengers that I could not leave my seat at the time. "If you are experiencing a medical emergency, please leave your light illuminated, but if you want clarification of what the captain just said, please turn your light off," I announced. All but one light went off; it was the same passenger, so,

I spoke to him through the PA because we were still bumping. He told me he really needed a drink. I explained it was not in his best interest or mine for him to have an alcoholic beverage at this time. I told him we would be on the ground shortly. As soon as I said that the plane took another drop. Some of the oxygen masks fell. Passengers were now overwhelmed. I called into the cockpit to inquire about the masks and was told it was most likely a malfunction because cabin pressure was not lost. I instructed the passengers who had their masks hanging down that they did not need them at that time. The captain came on the sound system and stated we would feel less turbulence shortly. We had already been in turbulence on and off for at least 45 minutes and this was only an hour and fifteen-minute flight. The baby was still crying. I know this is not what was supposed to happen during flight, but my instincts told me to get my CD player from out of my jacket pocket and play some music while holding the phone in announcement mold. For the life of me, I can't remember what songs played but it calmed the baby and the other passengers and gave me some relief as well. We made it through the turbulence and to our destination safely. As each passenger exited the plane, I wished them a blessed day, and in return they thanked me. The mother with the baby gave me a hug and thanked me for playing the music.

All of the passengers had exited the plane, with the exception of the passenger who kept requesting in-flight service. As he gathered his things, I wondered what he would have to say. He came closer to me and said, Thank you! I never had anyone tell me they had my best interest in mind." With that he exited the plane. The captain and the co-captain came out the cockpit. "That was a rough ride," the captain said. "How did it go?" I responded, "We managed, and our prayers were answered." Jokingly, the captain said, "Not bad for an overpaid waitress."

I shared this story because some people have said, when I advise them to live a healthier lifestyle that they are going to die from something. They don't think their *something DAY* is coming. This is my thought about the man on the plane. I believe he was someone who used alcohol to relieve stress or for self-medication. I can't say for sure. I feel like my heart spoke to his heart in a time of turmoil.

The next time you are eating at a restaurant and you know you struggle with eating healthier, when your server comes to your table, look at them as a vehicle to a healthier beginning. See them as someone who has your best interest in their hands. Be willing to go through the storm. Decide to die from *something* that is out of your undertaking. The turbulence experienced during the flight was out of my control, yet I did what I could to not bring more disorder to the situation.

The Brains Of The Operation

One day, my daughters, 10 and six at the time, were visiting their grandparents when they decided they would help their grandparents with chores around the house. At the time, their great grandfather (who was 86 years old) lived with my parents. My 10-year-old gathered her sister and cousins to give them a list of the chores they would do for the day. They started on the first floor of the house; cleaning the living areas (living room, family room and kitchen). They worked their way to the second floor, making the beds and cleaning the bathrooms. My ten year old, discovered the laundry wasn't done, so she took the laundry to the laundry room to wash. About this time, I called to check up on them. Here's how the conversation went:

10 year old: Mommy, we're helping grandmother clean-up.

Me: That's fantastic!

10 year old: Wait a minute, Mommy. I need to pour in the detergent.

Me: Wait a minute. Where is your grandmother?

10 year old: She went to the store.

Me: Who's there with you all?

10 year old: Papa Lee.

Me: Who's doing the laundry?

10 year old: I am.

Me: Honey, stop what you're doing.

10 year old: Mommy don't worry, Papa Lee is the brains of the operation.

Me: You're doing a great thing by helping out around the house, but wait until your grandmother gets back.

There are several parts of the brain: occipital lobe, temporal lobe, frontal lobe, cerebral cortex, cerebellum, hypothalamus, thalamus, parietal lobe, amygdala, hippocampus, and the mid-brain, just to name a few. The functions of the brain are: attention and concentration, organization, speaking (using expressive language), awareness of abilities and limitations, personality, mental flexibility, self-monitoring, inhibition behavior, motor planning and initiation, emotions, problem solving, planning, anticipation, and judgment. There are many schools of thought that encourage us to exercise our brains. We should intentionally do that daily. Amusingly enough the brain is not a muscle. For the purpose of this area we will focus on exercising your brain. The brain is the mother board of the body. Belief systems are passed down from one generation to the next. This can explain why you think the way you think and how you act or react to certain triggers in your life.

While our legacy is essentially based on our family experiences, I am advocating that just like the brain, there are many corridors a person can take to assure that they live a healthy lifestyle. Growing up without a blueprint to show how to manage your health can become a force of resistance, which can lead to trial and error. Although errors can build your mind and strengthen your decision making, it is helpful when you have a template that has been passed down from generation to generation. This can give you clear vision on how to navigate growth.

Having personal knowledge of what is important to live in optimal health is priceless. Ensuring you transfer information (i.e. physical attributes) about your ancestors is a way to empower the next generation so they can know how to live life to the fullest.

Living a healthy lifestyle starts in the mind. It's a mechanism that cognitive and behavioral action uses to encode the priority of what information is being stored. You may ask yourself a series of questions. For instance, what is a healthy meal to eat? How much of the meal should I consume? Do I have the knowledge and the finances to support this kind of lifestyle?

The CDC Second National Report on Biochemical Indicators of Diet and Nutrition, released in 2012, gives a better understanding of potential causes of deficiencies. The report used The National Health and Nutrition Examination Survey (NHANES) data from 2003-2006 for 58 indicators of diet and nutrition like vitamin D, iodine, and folate. For instance, overweight persons generally had lower nutrient levels. Based on body mass index, overweight persons had lower levels of vitamin B6 (13%), vitamin C (roughly 10%), vitamin D (roughly 8%), vitamin B12 (4%), serum folate (4%), and vitamin A and E (1%) compared to normal weight persons. Persons who reported consuming dietary supplements had higher levels of most nutrients. For instance, vitamin B6 (79%), vitamin C (roughly 30%), folate (24-36%), iodine (22%), vitamin B12 (21%), vitamin D (roughly 9%) and vitamin A (5%) levels were higher compared to non- dietary supplement users.

And be not conformed to this world; but be ye transformed by the renewing of your mind, that ye may prove What is that is good, and acceptable, and perfect, will of God. Romans 12:2 KJV

Am I My Brother's Keeper?

Our world is at the threshold of governing ourselves differently due to COVID-19. Researchers are searching our history to see if it can be a predictor, and then give us an answer on how to solve this contagious virus.

COVID-19 is a crisis around the world. It has certainly challenged each of us to look out for one another. Can you imagine what you do can directly affect your community? If we watched out for each other we would approach how we move about during this pandemic. Co-workers, friends, and loved ones, each one of us should wear a mask to help slow down the spread of this virus. The mask can help protect our most vulnerable population, our fellow woman, man, and child, our elderly loved ones, and those with underlying illnesses.

Let's take this same approach to our workplace. Most of

us know which of our co-workers have underlying health issues. Yet, we still celebrate milestones, promotions, and holidays with food that may not be favorable to someone with underlying life-threatening medical conditions.

I was told a story about a friend who had an annual adult beverage weekend party with his friends. One of the friends had a bad relationship with liquor and had gone to rehab in between the last adult beverage weekend event. The host of the party was the only one who knew about this guy's stint in rehab; rather than provide adult beverages he made smoothies, fruity non-alcoholic drinks, and ice cold water. His other friends wanted to know what was going on and why he wasn't serving alcohol. The host explained to his friends, without telling who it was, that someone at the party was struggling, and he wasn't going to make his friend's journey worse by tempting him.

Here is a story I want to share that personally happened to me. I have a good friend who I invited to go to lunch with me. It was a spontaneous request. She accepted my offer to pay for the meal and I sent her the menu ahead of time so she could choose what she wanted to eat. A few minutes later, she called to tell me there was nothing on the menu she wanted to eat. This friend is vegan(ish), but she will eat seafood. The restaurant I choose served sushi, raw veggies, and vegetarian sandwiches. I thought it was a great place to eat. However, she decided to bring her own lunch! I was impressed that she did not give in to a spontaneous event of eating out. Instead, she stuck to her own nutritional intake for that day.

Living a lifestyle that supports good health, and modeling that, does not limit your legacy to your biological family. Your legacy can include your work family, sports family, school family, and social group family. The answer to the question, "Am I my brother's keeper" might very well be *yes*.

By the time this book is published, I don't know if the statistics will be out to see how well our health has gotten due to the stay at home order. We are not able to participate in eating badly at work or picking up something quick to eat. I think, for the most part, we may be shockingly surprised that our bad eating habits away from home are a direct link to our eating habits while being social.

HOLIDAY/WORKPLACE SURVIVAL KIT MORE

TIPS ON SURVIVING SOCIAL GATHERING

Do pre-holiday planning. Decide ahead of time how you will handle the different events of the season. For non-festive days, plan healthy meals, and get some exercise every day.

Eat a snack before going to a party. Have yogurt or fruit, a few crackers with low-fat cheese, vegetables, or a skim-milk latte so hunger won't rule your choices.

Indulge moderately. No need to do without your favorite foods. Take small portions and eat slowly. That way you'll eat less and savor more. A small taste can satisfy your craving.

Let your eyes feast first. Before eating, see what is being served. If there are raw vegetables or plain seafood, start with those to take the edge off your appetite.

Avoid guilty pleasures you can have anytime, such as chocolates or chips. Go with seasonal favorites such as pie or cake. Enjoy, but keep portions small.

Stand far away from the buffet table. Once you've chosen your food, take your plate into another room and enjoy calorie-free talk with friends. Make one trip to the buffet and be selective.

Hold your drink in your right or dominant hand. If you are right-handed hold in right hand (left hand if you're a lefty). It will allow you to pause before you reach for food on impulse.

At a sit-down dinner, eat slowly. Put your silverware down between bites and chew thoroughly. Talk between bites so your meal will last longer. Split dessert with someone.

"If my people, which are called by my name, shall humble themselves, and pray, and seek my face, and turn from their wicked ways; then will I hear from heaven, and will forgive their sin, and will heal their land" II Chronicles 7:14 KJV

Build For Energy Or Made For Fat. Can't Do Both

We sometimes gain life in the way we give it away.

In the beginning of this book, I told you how much I enjoyed leaping and running around outside when I was a little girl. I learned jumping over branches was not going to be the hardest thing I ever had to get over. I tell you, when God commissioned me to write this book, this chapter was NOT going to be it. I had decided it wasn't necessary to air *everything*. Well, God said, if you believe you are forgiven, you will add this chapter. I thought I could write this book chronicling my childhood, adolescence, and then onto my age of doing better. I thought I could skip the growing up in my 20's part, but God held this book up until this chapter was written.

After adding this chapter, which I quickly completed, the book was done. I sent it to be copyrighted and the next day I had to hit the reset button again and learn how to "Grow the Health Up!"

Living my life by honoring my family has always been in the forefront of my movement in life. I recognized as I planted my steps through this life that I would bring my family's reputation with me. As a young, single woman I admit I made my share of poor choices and decisions. I made decisions that my young self would never have seen coming. The thought of it was unthinkable and I stood firm in judgment of those who would make such a decision. I was taught right from wrong. Living my parents' truths is how I started out in my adult life. I remained single until age twenty-five.

That's when I got married and had my first child, a child I didn't think I deserved. From the time I found out I was pregnant with my oldest living child, I was terribly anxious. I felt she would not make it to full term. Not because my health was poor, but because of the poor decisions I made, prior to this pregnancy, not to carry my pregnancies full term. I thought I would reap what I had sowed.

The first sign that I might lose my baby came when I was about eight weeks pregnant. My doctor told me my blood test revealed my baby could be born with birth defects. He wanted to know if I wanted to continue the pregnancy. I didn't give him an answer right away. After my husband and I talked about it first, we decided to go through with the pregnancy. I started researching different possible birth defects and began to plan for a child who would have it.

Seeing my beautiful baby's face when I gave birth was like seeing an angel. Since then, I have given birth to two more gorgeous daughters. Still, with each pregnancy, I was filled with anxiety. I didn't realize that 27 years later I still felt the wrath of God would come down on me, but then my twin granddaughters were born. I had to deal with the fact although I made poor decisions, I was forgiven years ago. I needed to forgive myself. As a Christian, I recognized that Jesus died on the cross for my sins. However, for a long time I believed there were levels to sin.

For instance, I used to believe telling a lie to keep from hurting a person's feeling versus a person who rapes and steals were two different levels of sin. I had a full circle moment as my faith walk matured and I grew up. I'm glad I know now that my sins are forgiven. I had to forgive myself for the bad decisions I made and will continue to make.

After a few years of marriage, I divorced and found myself single again. I was at the threshold of giving birth to my second born child. Growth and maturity aligned me with the insight that I wasn't going to have this moment define my life's purpose. I moved to my valley called Golden

Valley, Minnesota. Minnesota is where I began to heal, grow, and reconnect to my life's purpose. I moved to Minneapolis, Minnesota with one child in a car seat and the other one in my stomach. I drove 14 hours in a car that was brand new 8-10 years ago. Each time I stopped to fuel up or get a bite to eat, I had to put a liter of oil in the car. I was going to Minnesota to get the life God had planned for me and my children. I didn't have a job, but I knew my life from that point would forever change. This stage of my life, I was ready to live in my truth.

My children and I lived in a friend's basement in Minnesota for four months. If I ever needed clarity in my life, living in an unfinished basement definitely gave me understanding and quickly put a fire in my belly to do better. I want to say thank you to "Sharon." It was her kindness that allowed me and my babies to have shelter in her basement.

The first day I arrived in Minnesota, my sister-in-law told me about a position that had opened. The job listing was closing the next day, but I called and was able to secure an interview. I got a call back, had a second interview, and I was offered the job. I worked at Courage Center in Golden Valley, Minnesota for seven years. Seven is the number of completion. This was the vine that I used to earn my first college degree in Occupational Therapy. I earned two more degrees with the help of people God sent to me on this journey. Thank you to Saint Catherine's Single Parents Program, and to Karrie, Jean, Susan, Michael, Marlo and David. I'm thankful for the different grants I was able to obtain with their help. Without these people and these programs, my journey could have taken a lot longer.

Soon after moving to Minneapolis, I found a church home, Pilgrim Rest Baptist Church, and started attending on a regular basis. My girls started a Montessori pre-school. From there, I enrolled them in Christian elementary private schools. They have personal relationships with God. They became missionaries at a young age. Both developed as skilled pianists, accomplished dancers, and kind and giving girls. They have both earned their college degrees. They are productive citizens thriving in their careers with characteristics that we, as Americans, hold in adoration.

In life, we can either build for energy or for fat. When building for energy, at some point, we must have faith and believe that God is love, forgiveness, and all things that are good for us. Faith without works is dead. Living in good health and wellness takes active participation. It calls for forgiving yourself when you fall short. Just know that at a blink of an eye, you can make a decision to do better.

There was one occasion when I worked a second job at the airport as a ticket agent. This job afforded me the opportunity to travel the world with little to no money. After a year of being in the valley, I was able to purchase a better running vehicle. Before leaving Minnesota, after 10 years, I purchased a brand new car. I got married again to my Boaz. I am forever grateful to God for trusting me, and believing in me, although I did not always know this then, I surely know it now. God will never fail.

I was active in our church. I was an usher and this is where my health ministry began. I have remained faithful to the health ministry and ushering, no matter where we lived in the world. On any given Saturday, I could be found exercising my faith during my church ministry using my gifts to teach others how to become greater stewards over their temple. On Sunday, I was on my post, seating God's disciples during church service.

I have learned that there are people I am supposed to serve with my gifts, my talents, and my tithes. I volunteered at women's shelters and at elementary schools. In my valley, the most I earned from my job was $888 a month. I won't go into great detail of what that meant. What I will share with you is God blessed me. He was there with me daily. God provided for me and my babies and we did not lack for anything.

I wrote this chapter not just to bare my soul and to be transparent; it's more important than that. If there is a woman or man at the threshold of giving your life away, I want you to know you can be courageous. You are loved. You are an overcomer. God will send you help. I urge you to widen your vision. Take off your current lens. Like my mother used to say, hard is hard. I learned that I had to "Grow the Health Up" and start living a life of healthy living, not just for me but for my legacies (children, grandchildren...) to come. I do not stand in judgment of you or anyone. May peace follow you all the days of your life.

I had a picture of my girls glued to a mounted frame that I placed at the front door threshold in every apartment or house where we have lived over the last 10 years. Below their pictures I had the poem "Don't Quit" published by Edgar A. Guest, which predates 1921 and is now credited to John Greenleaf Whitter. I would read it and place my hand on that frame each time I walked out the house. Over the protector visor, inside my car, I had the poem "Footprints." I read it as I made it home with the girls safely.

DON'T QUIT

When things go wrong as they
sometimes will
When the road you're trudging
seems all up hill,
When the funds are low and the
debts are high
And you want to smile, but you have
to sigh,
When care is pressing you down a
bit,
Rest if you must, but don't you quit.
Life is strange with its twists and
turns
As every one of us sometimes learns
And many a failure comes about
When he might have won had he
stuck it out;
Don't give up though the pace seems
slow
You may succeed with another blow.
Success is failure turned inside out
The silver tint of the clouds of doubt,
And you never can tell just how
close you are,
It may be near when it seems so far;
So stick to the fight when you're
hardest hit
It's when things seem worst that you
must not quit

PSALM 10:17-18 KJV

17 Lord, thou hast heard the desire of the
humble: thou wilt prepare their heart,
thou wilt cause thine ear to hear:
18 to judge the fatherless and the
oppressed, that the man of the earth may
no more oppress.

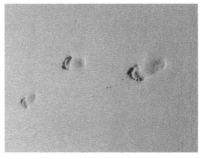

Photo by: Debra Duffy Footprints of Juanita,
Danielle, and Brianna

The main ingredient that keeps me steadfast is living a life of *fasting*. Fasting is an important part of my prayer walk, when seeking guidance from God. It may prove to be the change you are seeking.

Suggestions when building for energy and not fat:

1. Water/Fruit smoothies	1. Prayer/reading the word
2. Bananas	2. Pilates/Yoga/Meditation
3. Oats	3. Resistant Training
4. Greek Yogurt	4. Plyometric
5. Raisins	5. Walking
6. Nuts and berries	6. Zumba or Dancing

If I Only KNEW...I Would Have Moved FASTer

Most of you have heard about *fasting*, but may find it difficult to include it as part of your lifestyle. You know God is not a magician or a genie that grants wishes. A lot of churches use the *21 Day Daniel Fast*. The reason for the fast usually relates to a particular area in one's life that they would like to focus on to begin anew, to gain clarity, to have a closer and more intimate relationship with God, or perhaps to hit the reset button in their physical fitness and nutrition decisions.

Fasting can be achieved with a group of people who are fasting to gain the same thing or it can be followed through individually. For the purpose of this book, I am focusing on nutritional and physical health. Keep in mind, the spirit may lead me to other areas, just like with fasting. We may start out with our own agenda and quickly learn that God has a different assignment for us. Research has shown if you do not smoke, become addicted to recreational or over the counter drugs, and you do not engage in risky behavior, the following statement is true—50 is the new 30, 40 the new 20, and 30 the new 10 year old. Before you know it, the 20-year-olds are back to being infants. One may argue whether at 20 years old you could feel infantile (that's for another book). The idea our society has adopted that your biological age is not really your physical age, is not the best way to assure quality of life. I say, be a 50-year-old who acts like a 50-year-old but take care of your inside and outside like a healthy 30-year-old.

There is a billion dollar industry that caters to the notion *you can eat what you want*. You can *pay someone to cut it off or take it out*. We have adults at kid-friendly eating establishments eating processed cheese pizza, consuming liters of pop, and getting no exercise. Imagine, we have cartoon characters that are marketing to parents. A television commercial may say something like *"We have food for every age* or *"While your child plays, we have a salad you can eat,"* but most of the time parents are ordering salad, pizza, fries, and a diet pop to go with that shake.

I understand there are a lot of households juggling with both parents working outside the home. The kids are involved in paid activities outside of the home. Time becomes a concern for parents. It becomes easier to go to fast food places or eat out. Maybe consider not using a spoon or a fork approach. Eating a vegetarian, and maybe Mediterranean meal, this nutritional option you can eat with your hands. It is more optimal for our digestive system and shouldn't give us an upset stomach. This is the more favorable way to go.

The Christian journey is one that comes with giving, praying, and fasting. These three tiers of Christian faith are the three strands that can propel our walk as disciples. God giving us these instructions is what makes this standard of living normal. In the words of the late Pastor James E. Hill during one of his presentations, "The Bible clearly sets forth a supernatural element and a natural aspect concerning divine health. God has dietary laws governing the foods that should be eaten to maintain healthy physical bodies. Disease and illness would be rare if every bloodstream was pure, and the body was not full of waste materials and toxins."

Bible fasting is giving up specific foods and drinks for a designated amount of time. Praying and getting guidance from God as to how long, as well as the reason why you are fasting, is an intimate conversation that should be between you and the Lord.

29 And God said, Behold, I have given you every herb bearing seed, which is upon the face of all the earth, and every tree, in the which is the fruit of a tree yielding seed; to you it shall be for meat. Genesis 1:29 KJV

Fasting Is The Great System Equalizer

A few days of fasting annually can prove to be useful as it becomes a cleaning filter in the blood to eliminate harmful waste and toxins. H2O (Water) is an important part of the flushing process. Imagine, while you fast, you abstain from eating and drink water only. Look at the clearness of the water. Imagine your body being like a test tube in the lab. In the test tube there is debris and other substances. As you begin to fill the tube for three days with water, the color of the liquid begins to change. Your urine is made up of water. During fasting, your urine is a great indicator of what is happening on the inside of your body. It dissolves substances that help the body to eliminate poisons. Most of the time, when we eat a heavy fat-based meal, it takes a toll on our kidneys and slows down our digestive tract. We can begin to feel sluggish and sleepy. This is due to an increase in toxins, which can make it difficult to think and maintain your attention span.

Nothing measures up to fasting when it comes to a method of increasing elimination of waste from the blood and tissues. After not eating for two or three days, be mindful of your glucose level dropping because during this time the body is no longer using sugar for energy. The body is not able to make enough insulin during the fast. It begins breaking down its own fat and protein as a source of energy. This is commonly known as *ketone bodies*. The physiological pathways become important in the house cleaning stage. As the fast progresses, contaminated secretions or more suitably, retained waste, are thrown out of the body and your system becomes cleansed. Stored toxins are also released into circulation to be carried to the organs (i.e., kidneys, bowels, lungs, skin) and eliminated.

But, if we walk in the light, as he is in the light, we have fellowship one with another, and the blood of Jesus Christ his Son cleanseth us from all sin." 1 John 1:7, KJV

Time To Start The Conversation About The N Word

Let no man despise thy youth; but be thou an example of the believers, in word, in conversation, in charity, in spirit, in faith and in purity. Timothy 4:12 KJV

I heard a story about an executive who ran a successful top fortune 500 company. He was 34 years old, married, and had a five-year-old son. As one would imagine, the man was extremely busy. He had little leisure time to spend with his family.

One day, the executive was at home in his office working on a presentation for a huge account that his company was trying to close the deal on. Because of COVID-19, the executive had to work from home. His son, who rarely saw his father in his office, came into the room and asked his father if he would play football with him. His father told his son he would play with him when he finished his project. Ten minutes later, the son came back into his father's office and asked his father if he was finished. His father told him he was not finished yet and to give him an hour and he would come outside and toss the ball with him. As you might already be aware, most five-year-olds do not have a since of time so as you may have guessed, the son came back in the room minutes later. The executive began to grow frustrated with his son's interruptions. He saw a national geographic magazine on his desk. He thumbed through it and came across a picture of the world. He tore out the picture and ripped it into pieces and handed it to his son. He said to his son, "Take these pieces of the world and put it together. Once you have put all the pieces together in the correct places, bring it to me and we will go out and toss the football." The executive thought this should buy him at least an hour, but much to the executive's amazement, his son returned 10 minutes later with the pieces all put together. The executive said to his son, "I told you to put them in the correct places." His son replied, "Daddy, I did." The father took the paper from his son. It had tape all over the page to hold the pieces together. The father examined his son's work. To his surprise, it was correct. He sat back in his chair, picked his son up, and placed him on his lap. "How did you do that so quickly?" The son replied, "I flipped the paper over and I saw a picture of a family on the back of the paper. I figured if I put the family back right, then the world would be right." And with that, the executive got up, went outside, and tossed the football with his son.

I have lived abroad as well as in many states in America. I have researched how other people around the world maintain optimum health without reinventing the wheel. They listened to their ancestors and passed down those instructions which can be valuable to the next generation. The formula tends to be simple. Eat from the earth, plants and berries. Fruits are the staples essential to providing our bodies with the nutrients needed to complete activities of daily living. Just like the picture of the family, on the other side is a whole world of people and families who practice eating plant-based foods.

I am not a nutritionist, but I play one at home. Remember the conversations you had with your mother or grandmother about foods that are good for body parts (i.e., head, hair, nails, eyes).

- Fish is good for the brain. The mineral in zinc is found in fish and shellfish. Research shows even a little deficiency of zinc impairs thinking and memory.
- Vitamin E is good for the hair.
- Cantaloupe is good for your eyes. It contains beta carotene (which can reduce the chance of eye disease).
- Chia Seeds (11 grams of fiber recommended intake

for magnesium, manganese, and calcium).

- Garlic and onions are good for addressing flu and cold viruses.
- Blueberries fight the bacteria that causes diarrhea (great source of antioxidants).
- Bananas are a natural antacid. High in potassium, they soothe heartburn or gastric distress.
- Spinach is a good source of folic acid and iron.
- Apples are high in fiber, vitamin C, and have a number of antioxidants.
- Avocados are fruit loaded with healthy fats instead of carbohydrates. They are high in fiber, potassium, and vitamin C.
- Strawberries are high in nutrients and low in both carbohydrates and calories.
- Other healthy fruit choices are cherries, grapes, grapefruit, kiwi, lemons, mango, melons, olives, peaches, pears, pineapples, plums, and raspberries.
- Nuts: The forgotten nutrients in nuts, seeds, and peanuts that we sometimes forget about are magnesium and vitamin E.
- Almonds have vitamin E, antioxidants, magnesium, and fiber. Research shows almonds can help you lose weight, and help with your metabolic health.
- Coconuts are good fiber. Coconuts have fatty acids called medium-chain triglycerides.
- Walnuts are good fiber.

- Vegetables: Eating a variety of vegetables will increase your chances of getting your recommended nutrients.
- Asparagus is loaded with vitamin K.
- Bell peppers are good antioxidants and have lots of vitamin C.
- Moringa benefits and promotes hormonal balance.
- Broccoli is good fiber, loaded with vitamins K, C, and protein.
- Cucumbers consist mostly of water. Loaded with vitamin K.
- Kale is loaded with vitamins K, C , and fiber.
- Vegetables like artichokes, brussels sprouts, cabbage, celery eggplant, leeks, lettuce, mushrooms, radishes, squash, Swiss chard, turnips, and zucchini are all good sources for Vitamins K, C, and fiber.
- Grains like brown rice have fiber, vitamin B1, and magnesium.
- Oats are full of fiber called beta-glucans (a form of soluble dietary fiber strongly linked to improving cholesterol and boosting heart health).
- Quinoa is high in fiber and magnesium. Excellent source of plant-based protein.
- Ezekiel bread may be the healthiest bread on the shelf. It is made from organic, sprouted whole grains and contains several types of legumes.
- Beans, such as kidney beans and lentils, are a

good source of vitamins, minerals, and fiber.
- Ginkgo biloba contains powerful antioxidants, helps with circulation and heart health.
- Protein is essential for your body. Your body could not function without it. You need enough protein daily. Other than food sources, you should supplement your diet with a shake or bar as a midmorning grab and go or an afternoon pick me up. Whatever your preference, be certain to include enough protein every day.
- Water: You can go without eating for days, even weeks, but you cannot go very long without water. Every cell in your body is craving for the quenching effect of hydration. Revitalize your cellular strength, bring more life into your skin, and supply your body with organic minerals that protect it from disease and chemical imbalance with every drink of water. Drink alkaline water when you can.

Maintain Your Sugar Levels

When you eat foods higher on the glycemic index, your body feels the need to eat more food. However, the lower on the glycemic index it is the less likely you will continue to feel hungry after eating.

Minimizing the amount of junk food you eat is at the top of the label. That is why it is so easy to binge and continue to eat without thinking about it.

Glycemic index: A system that ranks foods on a scale from 1-100 based on the effect on blood sugar levels. You want to have staple foods in your diet. Most staple plant-based foods are derived from cereal such as wheat. Below are some staple foods.

- Wheat
- Rye
- Barley
- Maize
- Root vegetables
- Potatoes
- Yams

- Taro
- Cassava
- Dried Legumes
- Sago
- Fruits (Plantains)
- Fish/Salmon

Eat well and it will show from the inside out.

TIPS FOR CHOOSING HEALTHY FOODS AT RESTAURANTS

Look for the foods below on menus for lower calories, less solid fats (saturated/trans), and sodium.

Fast Food	
• Grilled chicken breast sandwich, no mayonnaise • Single hamburger, no cheese	• Grilled chicken salad with reduce-fat dressing • Low-fat or fat-free yogurt

Deli / Sandwich Shops	
• Fresh sliced vegetables on whole-wheat bread with low-fat dressing or mustard	• Turkey breast sandwich with mustard, lettuce, and tomato • Bean soup (lentil, minestrone)

Steakhouses	
• Lean and broiled beef (no more than 6 ounces) filet mignon, round and flank steaks	• Baked potato, no butter, margarine, or sour cream • Seafood dishes that are not fried

Chinese	
• Zheng (steamed) • Kao (roasted) • Shao (barbecue) • Light stir-fried in mild sauce	• Reduced-sodium soy, hoisin, and oyster sauce • Dishes without MSG added • Bean curd (tofu) • Moo shu vegetables, chicken, or shrimp • Hot mustard sauce

Italian	

109

• Lightly sauteed with onions, shallots, or garlic • Red sauces-spicy marinara sauce (arrabiata), marinara cacciatore, red clam sauce • Primavera (no cream sauce)	• Lemon sauce • Florentine (spinach) • Grilled (often fish or vegetables) • Piccata (lemon) • Melanzane (eggplant)
Mexican	
• Served with salsa, salsa verde (green chili sauce), or picante sauce • Topped with shredded lettuce, diced tomatoes, and onions	• Served with or wrapped in a corn or whole-wheat flour (soft) tortilla • Simmered with vegetarian chili or tomato sauce
Middle Eastern	
• Fava beans or chickpeas • Basted with tomato sauce	• Couscous (grain) • Rice or bulgur (cracked wheat)
Japanese	
• House salad with fresh ginger and cellophane (clear rice) noodles • Chicken, fish, or shrimp teriyaki, broiled in sauce	• Soba noodles (often used in soups) • Nabemono (soup/stew) • Tofu (or bean curd)
Indian	
• Tikka (pan roasted) • Cooked with or marinated in yogurt • Saag (with spinach) • Masala (mixture of spices)	• Tandoori (chicken marinated in yogurt with spices) • Pullao (Basmati rice)
Thai	
• Fish sauce	• Curry

CONCLUSION

"When we are born, we look like our parents, but at our death we sometimes look like our decisions."

When your friend says, "Girl, you look good. What do you do to stay that way?" You tell her you eat a plant-based diet, choose to drink a smoothie rather than pop, and exercise at least three to five times a week. She says, "I can't do all that." You say, "Grow the Health Up."

When your co-worker says you look great in that suit and asks what your secret is. You tell him you get at least seven to eight hours of sleep, eat six small meals a day, try to eat your last meal by 4:30 p.m., and engage in purposeful activity for at least 30 minutes every day. He says to you, "I can't start doing that today. It's all you can eat tacos during lunch today." You just say, "Grow the Health Up."

When your hair stylist says, "You always look so healthy and put together. Girl, how do you have time with your busy schedule?" You tell her you get up at 4:30 a.m., work out for 45 minutes, do yoga twice a week, and plan what you eat. She replies, " I don't have time to do that!" Just say to her, "Grow the Health Up."

When you have someone come into your life and they ask you to help them live a healthier lifestyle and they have tried to get on track, but they need a partner, try saying to the person, "*I'm here for you. I'm willing to go through this journey with you. I understand all too well my purpose in life, that I am accountable for those who seek my help. I know God has sent you my way. I suggest you read "GROW THE HEALTH UP."*

I pray that this book sheds some light on how our habits can go beyond ourselves. I pray that it helps you, me, and all of us to be responsible for others. Especially those who we haven't met.

Who I am just keep occupying different body shapes but my soul and spirit remains the same, in Christ Jesus.

About the Author

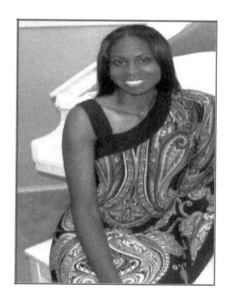

Debra McLemore Duffy is an entrepreneur (CEO) of her wellness firm. Her career path includes k-college level teacher, collegiate level basketball coach, and high school level track and field coach. McLemore Duffy has worked with wounded warrior heroes in TBI clinics, providing occupational therapy, which includes strategies or techniques to cognitive, behavioral or educational needs.

McLemore Duffy has 20 plus years of experience in

occupational therapy and 40 years of experience in teaching health and wellness to all mankind. She earned her undergraduate degrees in Occupational Therapy from The Saint Catherine's-Mpls, her undergraduate degree in Kinesiology and Master's in Education from University of Minnesota. She believes being in optimal health is the key to housing the Great That I Am, God. The best method to slow-down the prolonged onset of disease and illness is to first practice prevention.

As a military spouse to a husband who served 24 years in the military, she has worn many hats, but one consistent hat she wears is that of honoring God with all her heart.

14 But once the building of the temple was completed, God showed His divine approval by coming to dwell there in His glorious presence. 2 Chronicles 5:14 NIV

PHOTOS

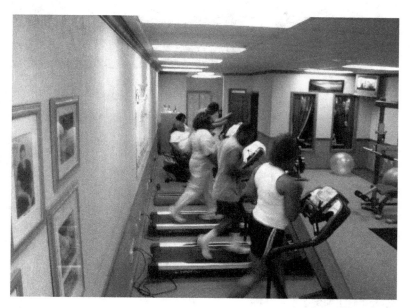

Photo by Debra Duffy

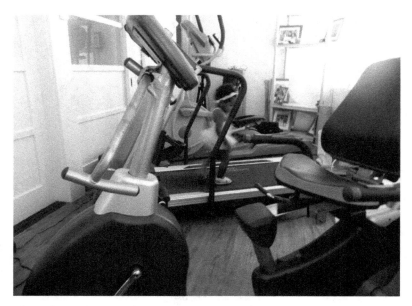

Photo by Debra Duffy

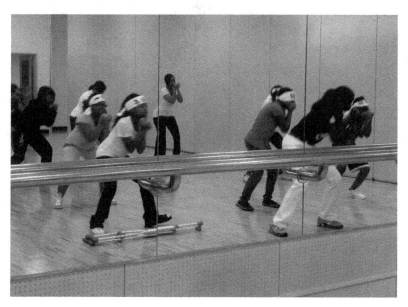

Photo by Debra Duffy

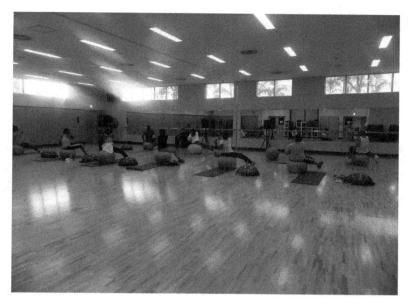

Photo by Debra Duffy

RESOURCES

Adapted from National Heart, Lung and Blood Institute (NHLBI), *Aim for a Healthy Weight; Maintaining a Healthy Weight On the Go-A Pocket Guide*, pages 14-18. http://www.nhlbi.nit.gov/health/public/heart/obesity/ AIM_Pocket_Guide_tagged.pdf

U.S. Department of Agriculture and U.S. Department of Health and Human Services. *Dietary Guidelines for Americans*, 2010, page 14. http://www.enpp.usda.gov/ dietaryguidelines.htm

RECIPES

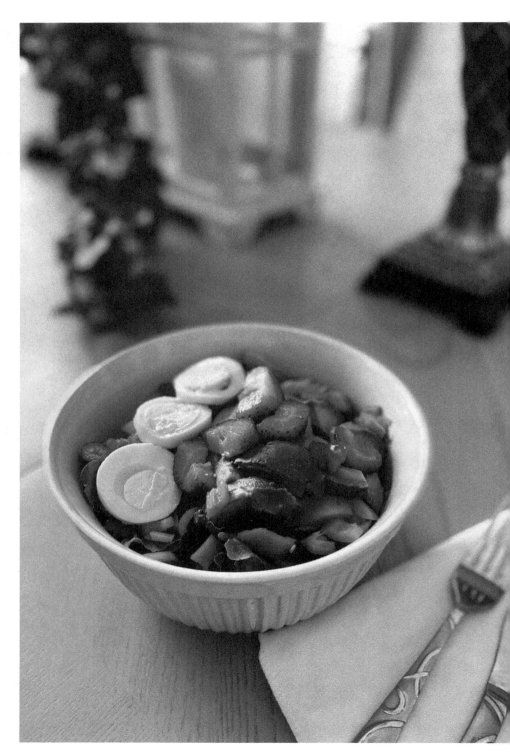

HOUSE SALAD

INGREDIENTS

- 3 cups of Organic Spring mix green leaves
- Avocados
- 2 Boiled eggs
- 3 Organic Cherry Size Tomatoes
- 4 Organic baby peppers
- Italian Castelvetrano Green Olives
- 1 cup Organic Granny Smith apple (green)
- 1 cup cucumber
- 1 tsp./5mil Pecans
- 1 tsp./5 mil Pistachios
- 1 tsp. /2.5 mil Pumpkin Seeds
- 1 tsp. /2.5 mil turmeric or ginger Dressing
- Extra Virgin Olive Oil(optional)

PREPARATION

Boil 1-2 organic non-caged brown eggs 5-10 minutes on medium heat. Once completely cooked, peel, cut, place in bowl. Cut up mixed greens, put into a bowl. Cut up tomatoes, bell peppers, green apple, and cucumber. Add to your bowl. Add 2-5 Green Olives, pecans, pistachios, pumpkin seeds, turmeric, and ginger. Add avocado. Add Extra Olive Oil for dressing (if desired). Enjoy!

Prior to preparing, testing or eating any of the nutritional suggestions, consult with your physician for guidance. This is intended for educational insight and not to replace your medical footprint. Do not use if you are allergic to any of the ingredients or if you don't know if you are allergic to any of the ingredients. Consult a trained medical professional to gather further information.

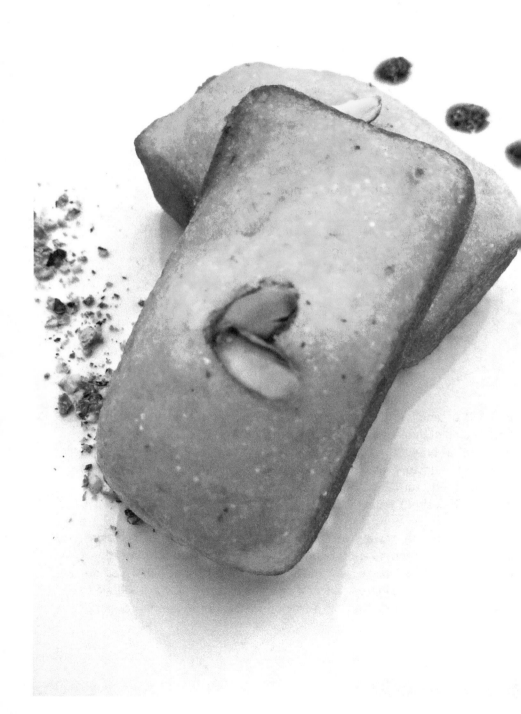

PISTACHIOS CORNBREAD

INGREDIENTS

- 4 tbsp. olive oil
- 1½ cups medium-grind corn meal
- 1 cup all-purpose flour
- 1½ tsp. baking powder
- 1½ cup of chopped pistachios
- 1 tsp. sea salt
- 2 eggs
- 1¼ cups milk, (more if needed)

PREPARATION

Preheat oven to 375 degrees. Put oil or butter in a 10-inch cast- iron skillet or in an 8-inch square baking pan. Place pan in oven. Meanwhile, combine dry ingredients in a bowl. Mix eggs into milk, then stir this mixture into dry ingredients, combining with a few swift strokes. If mixture seems dry, add another tablespoon or two of milk. When fat and oven are hot, remove skillet or pan from oven, pour batter into it and smooth out top. Return pan to oven. Bake about 30 minutes, until top is lightly browned, and sides have pulled away from pan; a toothpick inserted into center will come out clean. Serve hot or warm.

Prior to preparing, testing or eating any of the nutritional suggestions, consult with your physician for guidance. This is intended for educational insight and not to replace your medical footprint. Do not use if you are allergic to any of the ingredients or if you don't know if you are allergic to any of the ingredients. Consult a trained medical professional to gather further information.

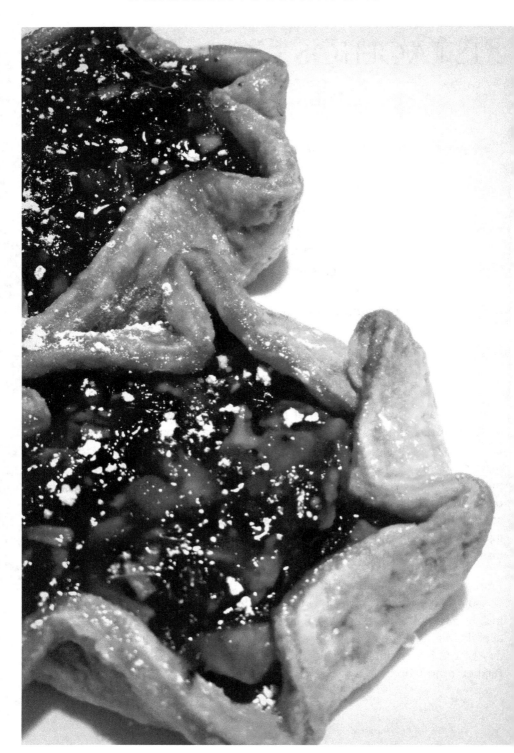

TART

INGREDIENTS

- 1 lb. berries (combination of cut up strawberries, blueberries, raspberries, and/or blackberries)
- 1 tbsp. cornstarch

PREPARATION

In a large bowl, combine berries, sugar, and cornstarch. Remove pastry from refrigerator and arrange berries on pastry, leaving about a two inch (5 cm) wide border. Gently fold edges of pastry up and over berries, pleating, as necessary. Make sure to seal any cracks in pastry. Bake for approximately 30 - 35 minutes or until crust is golden brown and juices are just starting to bubble and run out from center of tart. Remove from oven and place on wire rack to cool before serving. Serve with softly whipped cream or vanilla ice cream. Cover and refrigerate any leftovers. Makes about 6 - 8 servings.

Prior to preparing, testing or eating any of the nutritional suggestions, consult with your physician for guidance. This is intended for educational insight and not to replace your medical footprint. Do not use if you are allergic to any of the ingredients or if you don't know if you are allergic to any of the ingredients. Consult a trained medical professional to gather further information.

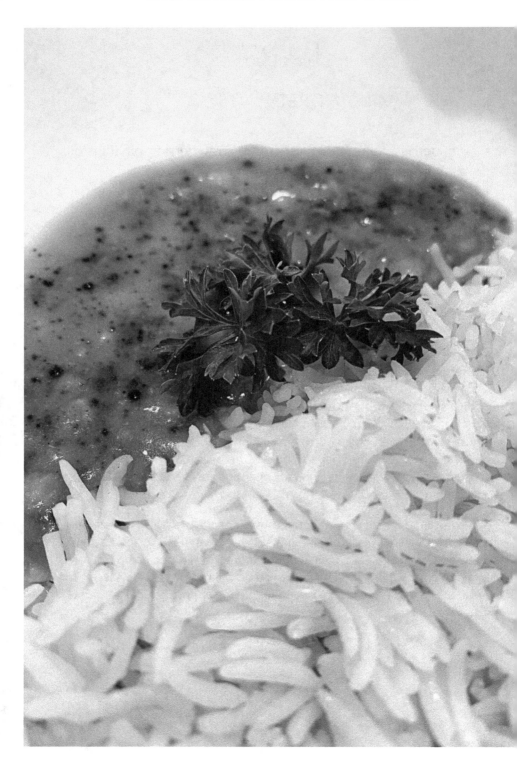

LENTILS AND RICE CURRY

INGREDIENTS

- 3 tbsp. melted coconut oil
- 1½ cups finely diced yellow onion
- 1 tbsp. finely minced garlic
- 1½ tbsp. finely minced ginger
- 2 tbsp. red curry paste
- 1 tbsp. yellow curry powder
- 1½ tsp. each: garam masala, paprika, ground coriander
- 1 tsp. ground cumin
- 3/4 tsp. turmeric

- Sea Salt and fresh ground pepper
- 1 can fire-roasted crushed tomatoes
- 1 cup green or brown uncooked lentils
- 1 can (14.5 ounces) coconut milk
- 3 cups chicken stock or broth
- 1/3 cup finely diced cilantro

- Optional: zest and juice of a lemon
- Optional: serve over cooked basmati rice

PREPARATION

Measure lentils and pick over to remove debris or shriveled lentils, and then thoroughly rinse with water. Add them to a bowl, cover in room-temperature water and let soak for 15-20 minutes.

SAUTE: Add 3 tablespoons butter or oil to a large pot. Heat to medium and oil is shimmering, add in the 1 cup onion, 1 tablespoon garlic, and 1 ½ tablespoon ginger. Cook and stir for 3-4 minutes. Add in 1 cup diced carrot. Cook, stirring occasionally for another 6-8 minutes or until everything is golden. Nothing should be overly browning or burning; if so, turn down the heat. While everything is cooking, measure out the spices.

SPICES AND TOMATOES: Add 2 tablespoons red curry paste, 1 tablespoon yellow curry powder, 1½ teaspoon garam masala, 1½ teaspoon paprika, 1 ½ teaspoon ground coriander, 1 teaspoon cumin, and 3/4 teaspoon turmeric. 1/4 teaspoon fine sea salt and ½ teaspoon ground pepper. Increase heat to high, stirring constantly, cook for 1-2 minutes or until very fragrant. Add tomatoes and reduce heat to medium. Stir and cook for 1 minute, scraping bottom of pot to release any browned bits.

LENTILS AND LIQUIDS: Thoroughly drain lentils. Add to pot along with can of coconut milk and 3 cups chicken or vegetable broth/stock. Bring to a boil and then reduce to gentle simmer. Cover with a lid and cook for 30 minutes, stirring every 8-10 minutes. Remove lid and simmer for another 5-8 minutes or until curry is thick and creamy and lentils are completely tender.

Prior to preparing, testing or eating any of the nutritional suggestions, consult with your physician for guidance. This is intended for educational insight and not to replace your medical footprint. Do not use if you are allergic to any of the ingredients or if you don't know if you are allergic to any of the ingredients. Consult a trained medical professional to gather further information.

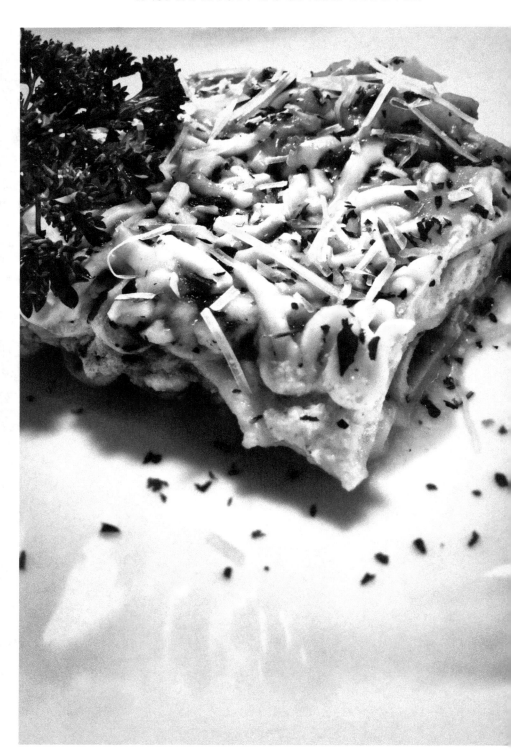

ZUCCHINI LASAGNA

INGREDIENTS

- 1 lb. ground turkey
- chopped onion
- cloves chopped garlic
- 1 can tomato sauce
- 1½ tsp. sea salt
- 1½ tsp. pepper
- 1 tsp. dried oregano
- 1 tsp. Italian seasoning
- ounces cottage cheese
- ½ cup grated parmesan cheese
- ounces zucchini or squash noodles (uncooked)
- ounces shredded mozzarella cheese

PREPARATION

Brown ground turkey, onion, and garlic in fry pan. Add tomato sauce, tomato paste, and dry seasonings. Cook long enough until warm. Spoon layer of meat sauce onto bottom of slow cooker. Add layer of noodles and top with cheese. Repeat with sauce, noodles, and cheese. Cover and cook on low 4 to 5 hours.

Prior to preparing, testing or eating any of the nutritional suggestions, consult with your physician for guidance. This is intended for educational insight and not to replace your medical footprint. Do not use if you are allergic to any of the ingredients or if you don't know if you are allergic to any of the ingredients. Consult a trained medical professional to gather further information.

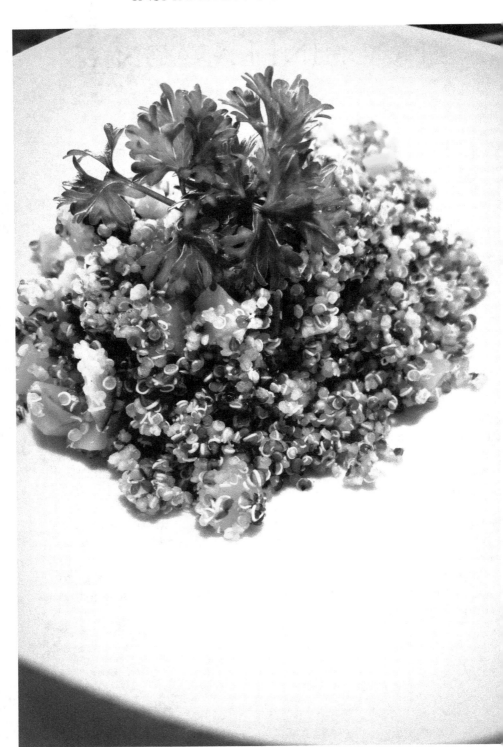

ISRAELI COUSCOUS

INGREDIENTS

- 1 lb. zucchini cut into pieces
- 1 lb. yellow squash cut into pieces
- 1 lb. peeled eggplant cut into pieces
- 1 large sweet red bell pepper cut into pieces
- 1 cup red onion sliced thin
- 3 tbsp. extra virgin olive oil
- ½ tsp. sea salt
- 1 tbsp. Greek or Mediterranean dried oregano
- 1 tsp. garlic powder
- ½ cup pitted and sliced Kalamata olives
- 2 tbsp. chopped fresh basil
- 2 tbsp. drained capers
- 1 tsp. freshly ground black pepper
- 1 pound Israeli couscous Vinaigrette, see below
- 1 cup crumbled feta cheese (optional)

PREPARATION

Preheat oven to 425 degrees. In a large bowl, place asparagus, zucchini, yellow squash, eggplant, red pepper, onion, oil, salt, oregano, and garlic powder. Mix to combine and pour out onto a sheet pan in a single layer. Roast vegetables for 10 minutes, flip and roast for 10 more. They should be slightly brown but still have some bite to them. Place vegetables back into large bowl and add olives, basil, capers and ground black pepper. In a large dry pan over medium high heat, toast couscous until slightly brown. Toss or stir often during browning so they don't burn. Bring 2 quarts of water to a boil with two teaspoons of sea salt. Add toasted couscous. Cook 8-10 minutes just until they are no longer hard but not too soft. (Al Dente) While couscous is cooking, make vinaigrette. Place all vinaigrette ingredients, except oil, into medium bowl and whisk. Slowly drizzle in oil while you whisk. Set aside. Once couscous is cooked, drain thoroughly in strainer and add hot couscous to roasted vegetable mixture. Toss slightly then add in vinaigrette. Toss again. Let sit for 30 minutes at room temperature so couscous can absorb the vinaigrette and flavors.

Prior to preparing, testing or eating any of the nutritional suggestions, consult with your physician for guidance. This is intended for educational insight and not to replace your medical footprint. Do not use if you are allergic to any of the ingredients or if you don't know if you are allergic to any of the ingredients. Consult a trained medical professional to gather further information.

CPSIA information can be obtained
at www.ICGtesting.com
Printed in the USA
LVHW082149151120
671787LV00049B/1693